▼

TELL
THE DRIVER

▼

Tell the Ⓞ Driver

▼

A BIOGRAPHY OF ELINOR F.E. BLACK, M.D.

▼

Julie Vandervoort

University of Manitoba Press

© Copyright Julie Vandervoort 1992
Published by University of Manitoba Press
Winnipeg, Manitoba R3T 2N2

Printed in Canada
Printed on acid-free paper ∞
Design: Norman Schmidt

All photographs courtesy of Fred Black unless indicated
otherwise.

Cataloguing in Publication Data

Vandervoort, Julie, 1958-
Tell the driver
Includes bibliographical references and index.
ISBN 0-88755-157-2
1. Black, Elinor F.E. (Elinor Frances Elizabeth),
1905-1982. 2. Gynaecologists - Canada - Biography.
3. Obstetricians - Canada - Biography. I. Title.
R464.B42V36 1992   610'.92   C92-098167-4

This book has been published with the assistance of the
Canada Council.

Contents

to Marc

Acknowledgements

TO FRED BLACK, executor of Elinor's estate, and to Anne Black, I express my warmest thanks and deepest gratitude. Four years is a long time to put up with regular visits, papers dragged out again and again, constant questions and requests. But the questions always received thoughtful answers, the atmosphere was always conducive to a free and open exchange of ideas and the self-invited guest was always offered a meal. It was a pleasure to work with you. My thanks also to *all* the Black family members who searched through old letters and their own memories and took the time to write it all down and send it to me. You made a real and valuable contribution to this book.

To my own family, and friends, the four years has undoubtedly seemed interminable. There are no words to describe the generosity of friends and family who accompany a writer through the turmoil and crises of a first book. My heartfelt thanks to: my sister Karen, who patiently coaxed my computer keyboard and screen into giving me one more chance to learn the program, and who so often got me back to work with love, sympathy and encouragement; James, who asked and listened and understood; my mom, Fay, and my sister-in-law, Peggy, who searched out medical articles and shared their knowledge; my brothers and father. To my friends, who laughed and helped and commiserated and suffered through endless Elinor stories and still stayed my friends and still kept believing in the book — your support meant, and means, more than I can say. My love, admiration and equally heartfelt thanks.

To the people of Winnipeg. The doctors and nurses, the librarians and archivists, the grant administrators, the friends and former patients of Dr. Black's and virtually everyone else I met or spoke to in Winnipeg exhibited such tremendous go-getting, problem-solving generosity of spirit that I was almost bowled over. My thanks to all, with special mention to Audrey Kerr and Natalia Pohorecky of the Medical Library, University of Manitoba, and to Dr. Dave Stewart and his wife, Ruth, of Killarney, Manitoba.

To the Ottawa women's writing group — this book wouldn't have happened without you.

Finally, I wish to acknowledge the help of Richard Holden, program officer at the Canada Council, and Patricia Dowdall, director of the University of Manitoba Press. Throughout this occasionally crazy-making project, thank you for those moments of extra humanity, courtesy and faith.

The author gratefully acknowledges the support of the Explorations Program of the Canada Council, the Paul H.T. Thorlakson Foundation, the Manitoba Heritage Federation, the T. Glendenning Hamilton Research Grant Program and the Ontario Arts Council.

▼

TELL
THE DRIVER

▼

One

FAMILY PLAYERS

▼

Dear Daddy,
I am sending this little letter all by myself. No one helped
me. (Elinor, age 7, letter in mother's handwriting.)

ELINOR WAS ONLY THREE DAYS OLD when a crisis abruptly forced her mother's attentions away from the newborn. Polio had just struck down Elinor's sister Charlotte, and Margaret Elizabeth McIntosh Black did not want to lose another daughter. She had lost two already: Dora, at two months, and then Jeannie, at four months, six days. Now Charlotte, not yet three, was fighting for her life, her diaphragm and legs seized by the dreaded "infantile paralysis."

There was almost nothing anyone could do to help. It was 1905; no one knew how polio was transmitted. For years afterward, the family believed that the disease was carried into the house on the big black cape worn by the maternity nurse who had come to assist at Elinor's birth. Assigning blame, however, was small comfort when there was no treatment. In this epidemic, as in those to follow, some children caught polio and others didn't; of those who did, some lived and others died.

Charlotte lived. (That fact wouldn't have surprised anyone who later had any experience with her indomitable will.) It was years before she could walk, and she never laughed out loud again — her diaphragm was permanently damaged.

In later years Elinor seemed almost proud, in a mocking kind of way, of her early introduction to independence. She once wrote to a friend, "I never got *bonded*; . . . mother, with the very ill 3 yr old, had no time to go parading around with me like a neat goose with her gosling."[1] From the available evidence, it appears that Elinor never did bond with her mother. Their relationship was neither warm nor involved, largely, it seems, because Elinor preferred it that way. It suited her better to cherish the idea that she could do everything herself, without any parental help. For intimacy and love, Elinor bonded to Charlotte, instead.

The relationship between the two sisters began in a highly charged atmosphere of anxiety and emotion and the feelings that connected them remained intense and powerful all their lives. For decades they were conspirators and pals, but eventually their interdependence and possessiveness of each other caused serious problems.

Elinor's first few years were spent watching Charlotte being wheeled around in a specially built pram. Charlotte gradually relearned to walk, but she fell so often that she wore a "bumping bag" — a bonnet stuffed with woolen socks — on her head. All this made the two girls seem more equal, closer in age. They were a team. Charlotte was older and knew more, and Elinor could be Charlotte's legs. Elinor had a sunnier, more mischievous disposition and her determination to "get around" their parents kept her older sister laughing heartily, albeit noiselessly.

There were also two older siblings in the family: Marjorie

and Donald. Details of Elinor's early years can be found in a rather reverential biography Donald wrote of their father, Francis Molison Black, known to family members as Frank. Donald recorded that at the time of Elinor's birth, the Black family was living in Nelson, British Columbia. The area was booming because of gold and silver, especially silver. It was rumoured that one mine alone, the Silver King on Toad Mountain, had attracted investment of over $2 million. Nelson started to regard itself as a very modern city with a great future.[2]

It must have been a fine place to be district manager, as Elinor's father was, of P. Burns and Co. Pat Burns was a millionaire cattle rancher, a founder of the Calgary Stampede and president of a meat-packing company that would gain international recognition by the First World War. With Frank working for Burns, the Black family could afford a Chinese servant, described as "pigtailed and felt-soled," and a summer home three miles east of town on Kootenay Lake. From here, in late spring, Frank would row the older children to school and himself to work.

In January 1909 Frank was promoted to company treasurer and he moved to head office in Calgary. There, he was in constant contact with Burns, a man Frank admired as someone who practised "restraint and modesty" and who generally "had himself well in hand."[3] Margaret and the children followed in July, and, according to one family friend, the servant was probably just as glad to see the last of them. By all accounts Margaret was an exacting — some say obsessive — housekeeper, and Margaret herself told the story of the servant turning away from her muttering "stinkum lady" before attempting to redo a task to meet her standards. The epithet caused great glee among the children, who insulted each other with it at every opportunity.

Once in Calgary, Margaret was well set up in a spacious

house that Frank had had built. The home featured six bedrooms (one for the maid), three fireplaces and ultra-modern central vacuuming. All that may have helped Margaret keep order domestically, but outside, the city was bustling, hustling and chaotic.

Donald writes that when they arrived in town the hitching posts on Eighth Avenue were just starting to come down, and the city's first skyscraper — the six-storey Grain Exchange Building on Ninth and First — was going up. Frank's office was also on Ninth, one block from the King Edward Hotel, an establishment that boasted the longest bar in Canada.

James H. Gray, in his chronicle of western wickedness entitled *Red Lights on the Prairies*, describes Calgary before the First World War:

> [Calgary's] building permits doubled and redoubled by the year, from $2,400,000 in 1909 to $20,000,000 in 1912.... By-laws by the barrel-ful were going onto the books.... New sanitary regulations had to be enforced. Cows and pigs running loose had to be impounded. People accustomed to tossing trash in alleys had to be reprimanded.... Chinese laundries had to be forced to stop dumping their tubs in ditches. The automobile was having such an impact that a whole new body of street regulations had to be enforced by a new breed of policeman — the traffic cop.[4]

There were still more social problems. Spitting was such a grave concern that the *Calgary Herald* ran a front-page editorial demanding the police enforce the by-law forbidding it. But it was drinking that really topped the list. In 1914 there were over 2,550 arrests for drunkenness and vagrancy.[5] Inevitably there was a reaction.

Gray describes the Protestant churches as working "both sides of the street" in their desire to bring about prohibition. The Total Abstinence League had their speakers and self-evident program, and the Anti-Treating League had theirs.

This latter campaign attracted less resolute souls who had only to pledge not to accept free drinks or treat friends to any.[6]

It's fairly certain that Elinor's father, a deeply religious Presbyterian and stern teetotaller, would have thrown his lot in with the first group. As he demonstrated many times, there were no half-measures when it came to principles and morals. In fact, Calgary's rowdiness may have been a factor in his decision to remove his family from its influence. But whatever his view of Calgary's charms, it was time for all the children to learn something of their Scottish heritage, and to this end the family moved again, to Edinburgh.

From Donald's account, it appears the family spent the summer of 1912 together, travelling across Canada, sailing from Montreal and then taking short trips in Scotland from their headquarters at Grandma Black's place in Perth. By September Margaret and the children were installed in a furnished house in Edinburgh. Donald went to George Watson's College, the girls to the corresponding Ladies College. Frank went back to Calgary and didn't see the family again until the following summer.

It would be interesting to know how Margaret felt about this latest move and separation. She wasn't a Scottish immigrant like Frank, although she did have a Scottish background, and it wasn't her roots they were tracing. It's not easy to find evidence of her true feelings; her presence seems almost erased from the picture — just like in Elinor's independent-minded letter to her father where the little girl claimed, not quite truthfully, that no one had helped her.

Frank, Donald and Elinor were all, to varying degrees, good correspondents, memoir writers, diarists and biographers, but little mention of Margaret is found in any of the material they left. Donald's account carries this description of his mother, written by Frank before they were married: "I certainly admire her as the best specimen of a good, well-educated woman that I have met, not withstanding the fact that she has spent all her life in the West and neither plays nor sings, while with it all there is a strong backbone of common-sense derived from ancestors in Strathspey."[7] A few of Margaret's letters did turn up, probably because they are mainly about Elinor (who kept and recovered extensive records on herself).One letter mentions Frank's work habits: "I am afraid you have been going at too great a rate for some time"; it ends with a very interesting question — "What do you think of the suffragettes now? Are they not fierce?"[8]

In a letter dated a few months later, Margaret reported to Frank that she returned home from a suffragist meeting and Elinor greeted her with, "Did you learn how to smash windows and houses, Mother?"[9]

That particular meeting was held at the home of the Pagan sisters, relatives Elinor later described as "some of grandmother's hundreds of first cousins." Frank called them "queer" but "people of understanding." One of the sisters, Isabelle, had recently published a complex analysis of religion and astrology. It became immensely popular and went through five editions.[10] One day, Isabelle Pagan cast Elinor's chart. Her predictions were astute, one of them being Elinor's future "guardianship of those weaker or more helpless" than herself. Pagan also divined devotion to profession, strong love of principles, tenacity of purpose, fulfillment through "teaching or preaching" and a desire to see "everyone living sensibly and healthily, without either luxury, or want." What isn't written in the chart, although the astrologer might have seen it, is that Elinor absorbed something of the suffragists' struggle. She was growing up as determined as they not to be denied, on the basis of gender, any place or privilege she felt was hers.

What *did* Frank think of the fierce suffragettes? He didn't

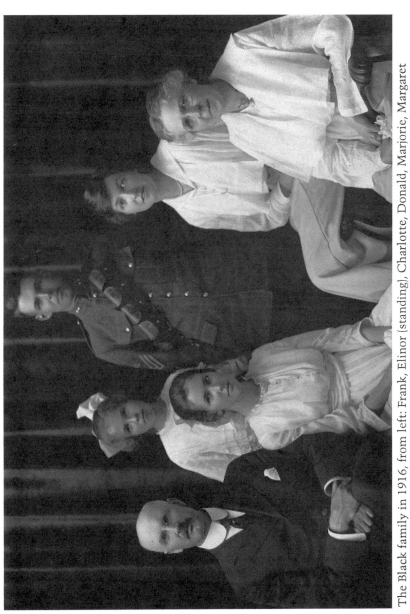

The Black family in 1916, from left: Frank, Elinor (standing), Charlotte, Donald, Marjorie, Margaret

discuss it with his seven-year-old daughter, but he did write to her, and his letters were carefully preserved in Elinor's scrapbook.

Despite the series of long separations from his children, no one could accuse Frank of being an indifferent father. His letters to "Dear Wee Elinor" are warm, comical and loving. He asks her if she can swim across the bath yet and whether she has heard the yellow bird singing "bread and butter but *no* cheese." He carefully put together picture-story letters. When Elinor boasted that she was sending replies all by herself, he teased her with — "What am I going to do? Here's my little baby writing letters all by her lonesome! But she can't be a baby any more if she is doing so! Then, *where* is my baby? I will have to put up a sign." He sketched a front lawn with a sign on it saying "Lost. One Baby Girl. Used to have yellow curls. Large reward."[11] Elinor loved that letter and made sure to revert to using "Your Loving Baby" as her sign-off when she answered it.

Elinor's letters are also comical. She wrote, "I was glad to see my old home again in the picture and my own, dear Daddy with his lead pencil hair. . . . Good night, Daddy. I love you." In another one she said, "Uncle Jack sent me 10 shillings for a Christmas card. Don't you think that was kind? I think I will get a dear wee muff and fur." On a less personal note, she informed her father that "[explorer] David Livingstone would be 100 years old today. He died on his knees before his bed with his candle burning and his Bible open."[12]

At times a plaintive note crept into these letters. Learning to play tennis with a carpet-beater racquet, eating porridge with a lace-capped grandmother and learning Highland dances were not enough to distract her from missing her father. Margaret described a little girl with a contagious laugh, a child "simply bubbling over with spirits" who investigated "all trees and flowers with joy."[13] But Elinor showed another side of herself to Frank. She wrote, "It isn't long until we go home!" She told him, "If you were here I'd give you a bear hug." In one of the final letters she said, "Mother gave me my bible at Christmas — I read out of it with Mother nearly every night. I will be glad to see you when I get home. I certainly wd not like to stay another year. . . . I will be very glad when I get home to Canada and *you*." (*"So will I,"* wrote Margaret in the margin.) Elinor ended the letter with, "I think you will know me."[14]

Clearly it was time to go back.

Frank came to collect his wife and children in the summer of 1913 but the family was not to remain together long. Margaret and the two youngest girls returned home, but the parents decided that the two elder siblings would have another year of Scottish education. Donald went to boarding school and Marjorie moved in with a widow and went to day school. By the time the teenagers headed for Canada the following August, the war had begun.

The First World War did not immediately disrupt the lives of the Blacks. Frank kept working for Pat Burns. Elinor was still writing self-possessed letters, using the very grown-up signature "Elinor F.E. Black." In one note, sent to Donald a few months after she returned to Calgary, she says, "I hope you are well. I am well. But I have a touch of growing-panes [sic]. But when I have them they aren't very bad and that I am thankful for."[15]

Elinor was being eased through her growing pains with deportment classes and art lessons. She was taught to carry her height well, but all she learned about art at this stage was how to avoid hard lines when applying water-colour washes. Art lessons in Winnipeg would have more of an impact but that would come later. For present, Calgary schools still had something to say about Elinor's character development, starting with the *Perpetual Exercise Book*.

Aptly named, this book provided every school child with a lengthy list of exhortations and instructions. Students were expected to sort out exercises of permanent value at the end of each term and file them away for future reference. They were also instructed to make maps of the school ground, town, school district, river, railroad and any excursions they went on. They were advised to collect stamps, and the stories of the struggles of the first settlers, including maps of the countries they came from. Another task was recording the weather, the length of the winter and the "opening" of spring. While the students were at it, they could estimate their rates of walking. And list the books or stories they read, noting main characters and names of authors. Monitoring newspapers for articles on famous writers was deemed a worthy activity. So was cutting out pictures of prominent men.

The concept of prominent *women* obviously hadn't quite made it into the curriculum. However, the reality of such women had entered the schools in the form of female medical inspectors. Dr. Lillias Cringan-MacIntyre and Dr. Geraldine Oakley were two such inspectors holding regular clinics in the public schools. It must have been fascinating for the young, ambitious Elinor to meet them. Women doctors! That would have been something worth thinking about. At the least, what they were doing looked like an alternative to housekeeping, something Elinor hated and learned to dodge by offering to do Donald's former jobs.

Years later, in an interview, Elinor credited Dr. Oakley and Dr. Cringan-MacIntyre with "firing her resolve" to be a doctor.[16] Their influence was Calgary's major legacy to Elinor — along with a lifelong dedication to collecting, sorting and recording the evidence of her own senses.

Winnipeg, the city Elinor later called "my sphere," was on the horizon, but the war was delaying her arrival there. The war had come closer to the Blacks. Donald had joined the

Canadian Expeditionary Force. Frank had resigned (on a matter of principle, Donald writes, regarding some financial policies) from Pat Burns' company and had been asked to serve on the War Time Food Control Board in Ottawa. Before he went, Frank, as president of Calgary's Board of Trade, gave a speech before six thousand people at a rally for the Patriotic Fund.[17] Author Francis Marion Beynon vividly captured the mood of such crowds in her contemporary novel, *Aleta Dey*. She described the "even tramp of troops" in the city streets, the morning bugle and the uneasy emotional mix of excitement and horror:

> What days those were! An extra every half-hour! War maps in every hand! A half mile towards Paris — gloom for two days! A great ship sunk — gloom for a week! Our hearts were sensitive to suffering then and the death of a hundred thousand men meant something to us. The blood reeked in our nostrils.[18]

Responding to their respective calls of duty, Frank left for Ottawa and Donald headed to Halifax. Donald shipped out only a few days before the Harbour collision of two ships, one loaded with munitions, caused the most devastating man-made explosion the world had yet seen.[19]

Margaret may have been worried sick, thinking about Donald's narrow escape, and lonely, with both her husband and son thousands of miles away. Elinor, though, was not entirely unhappy. Strong and athletic, it was logical that she step into Donald's shoes, even as young as she was. Charlotte wasn't physically able, and Marjorie was as dedicated to running a perfect household as Margaret. By default as much as by choice, it fell to "Babe," as they often called Elinor, to shovel snow and fix doorbells. She had a knack for the latter, and infinitely preferred the former to handstitching shirts for Donald, a task she detested.

Elinor resented Donald's unassailable status as eldest,

only boy and soldier. She sarcastically called him "the white-haired boy." At the same time, she was desperate for him to approve of her, or even notice her. She threw herself into proving that she could do the job at hand as well as Donald — or better. She had time to perfect this role; the household remained women-only for more than two years.

Elinor and her mother and sisters moved to Winnipeg in May 1918. Frank had a new job there as treasurer of United Grain Growers Limited, a farmer-controlled cooperative that operated hundreds of grain elevators. He had started the previous September, but Margaret and the girls didn't arrive until nine months later. This may have been because of the war, or because, as Donald's account has it, the first few months in Winnipeg were difficult for Frank as he sorted out the endless complications of the expanding company.

The influenza epidemic may have been another consideration. As mysterious a killer as polio, the 'flu virus seemed intent on sapping the last bit of strength and morale from communities already devastated by war losses. Over 13 thousand cases were reported in Winnipeg alone, and each day saw another 20 or 30 people dead. Schools and churches closed down for weeks, public assemblies were banned. The Children's Hospital housed many infants and young children who weren't sick but whose entire families had taken seriously ill or died. Authorities didn't know where else to put them.[20]

Frank finally transferred his family anyway, perhaps reasoning that no place was truly safe from the deadly virus, and no one knew when the situation would ease. Shortly after arriving in Winnipeg, Elinor caught it. Once again, the parents struggled with the anguish of not knowing the cause or cure, knowing only that young, healthy adults seemed to be hit first and hardest in this vicious epidemic. Should one try oil of cinnamon drops? Long walks in the fresh air? Nose and mouth masks? Who knew? But Elinor pulled through, making a complete recovery. The luck of the draw.

When Elinor came to Winnipeg she was almost 13. In her retirement years, she decided to write a sort of autobiography and she started it here — at the junction of Winnipeg and adolescence. She called the 100-page manuscript "The Professor and His Wife" and it was intended as a tribute to two of the most pivotal characters in her life. In the process of describing Arthur Stoughton, founder of the University of Manitoba's School of Architecture, and Florence, his wife, Elinor wrote her own story. This is how it begins:

> He was the Professor of Architecture and she sang alto in the church choir. That is all I knew about these new friends of my parents when I first met them as a child of twelve. She was three or four inches taller than he and the difference in height was exaggerated by the long braids of dark hair coiled on top of her rather small round head, which, in turn, was usually surmounted by a large hat, the mode in 1918. I thought she looked like an ostrich because the small head was held very erect on a long neck rising from narrow shoulders; her hips were disproportionately wide, her thigh bones very long, and the lower legs tapered to very thin ankles. Her face was nice: a flat profile with an abrupt small nose, a wide smiling mouth with white even teeth, and beautiful dark brown eyes with heavy lashes. If one were sitting alongside of her she had a habit of turning her whole upper body to look at one instead of just turning her head, a movement that was rather intimidating until one became used to it. Years later when I saw Disney's "Fantasia" with its ballet of ostriches, my thoughts went back to my early impressions of Donna [Florence].[21]

Elinor turns the same searching camera's eye on "Pater," Arthur Stoughton, and records another bird — a toucan with black hair and moustache, a heavy arched nose and strange awkward hands with the thumbs set far back from the palms, "like a monkey's." Infinitely kind-hearted and almost equally impractical, the Stoughtons appointed themselves Elinor's first set of patrons. It proved a mixed blessing.

And what did they see, these two exotic ornithological types, when they looked at Elinor? They would have seen a tall, gangly adolescent so skinny she could make a skirt out of one leg of her father's pants (using the other leg for fashionable side panels). Her hair was golden blonde but it wasn't being shown to best advantage at the moment. In an attempt to leave her babyish "Dutch" haircut behind her, Elinor agreed to have it tortured back into two pigtails at the earliest possible length. No hair hanging about the face in Margaret's household. Elinor learned to stop chattering when her mother or Marjorie did her hair; she was afraid her mouth wouldn't close again, the pigtails were so tight. And that wouldn't be too good, because she had very obvious braces.

"Delightful," thought the Stoughtons. "Enchanting! Exactly the little girl we would have wished for ourselves." They must have thought this, because they went to Elinor's parents and earnestly tried to adopt her. That was typical of the Stoughtons' other-worldliness, and lack of understanding of how the real one functioned. It's amusing to picture a solid friendship developing between these naïve artists and the strict, sober Blacks but that is what happened. Denied permission to adopt Elinor formally, they had to settle for calling her "Sweet Childe," which they did all their lives, and teaching her to call them "Donna" and "Pater." They spoiled and defended her — and took endless photos of her.

Elinor referred often to the photography sessions when she wrote this memoir; sometimes the tone is impatient and sometimes it seems distressed. The early photographs are romantic portraits of girlhood and "sylvan" studies of Elinor and Charlotte by the river. The later photos raise a few questions, even an eyebrow. Elinor described how the sessions began:

Dressed in the most filmy dresses that our thrifty and sensible ward-
robes contained, we repaired on sunny Saturday afternoons to the
river bank for what proved to be trying and tiring sessions. Pater
would pose us perilously among, on, and under artistically leaning
tree trunks, walk off a few paces to study the effect and the lighting,
come back to readjust an arm or a leg or the hang of a dress, and walk
off again. After two or three such excursions, the camera would be
set up, the square of black velvet arranged with difficulty, because of
the awkwardness of his hands, over his head and the camera and the
process of centring us upside down on the viewing plate would begin. This took some time and was inevitably interrupted by a breeze
blowing up the corners of the black velvet.[22]

Naturally the two girls thought this was quite funny but
out of genuine affection for Pater they tried not to laugh or
show they were bored by the whole business. Respect for
your elders and betters was highly prized by the Blacks and so
was modesty. Vanity wasn't. So the photos, some of them
beautiful (Elinor called them "acceptable"), were kept in a
plain brown envelope and never hung.

Charlotte is not in many of the photos with Elinor, but
when she is the closeness of the two sisters is obvious. Their
attachment thrived despite the fact they were becoming very
different people. Two sources — their letters to Santa Claus
and Elinor's autograph book — show how their values were
diverging.

Charlotte's letter to Santa begins by briskly reminding
him of his duty — "Dear Santa C.: The time for you to pay
your yearly visits again." She then went on to ask for presents
for Donald, Marjorie and Elinor; she put herself last. Charlotte also asked for something "that will help make things for
the poor and two shillings to help the poor old men and
women."[23]

Elinor could not match her sister in virtue and self-
sacrifice and she made only a passing attempt at it. She
started off properly subdued with "Dear Santa Claus — This

▼ 17 ▼

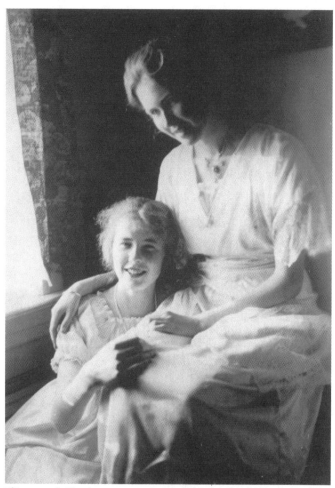

Elinor and Charlotte, Stoughton photo, 1921 (Department of
Archives and Special Collections, University of Manitoba)

Christmas things being so expensive I don't want many presents and of what I do want I expect to get only one thing." But her irrepressible enthusiasm took over: "Voici my list. A *Waterman's* self-filling, clip-cap fountain pen. A pair of nice warm mittens, a new pair of stays, a year's subscription to the *Popular Mechanics*, a *Canadian Girl's Annual*, 1920 edition, a red ribbon and tie, and if I got a watch I wouldn't throw it away." As Elinor glanced over her letter she may have felt a little stab of remorse. Did it sound excessive and greedy, despite her opening disclaimer? She hastened to let Santa know she had written it on the scrap piece of paper her mother had partially used to write Charlotte's get-out-early note. "Thus," she pointed out, "I am saving a piece of good writing paper."[24]

While Charlotte's goodness was a bit on the stern side, Elinor probably found it quite comforting. She liked to rebel but she also liked to have firm, fixed standards to rebel against and this was something her siblings and parents could provide in abundance. Charlotte, in fact, would later have herself tested in college by a psychologist offering "intelligence tests" and learn that her role in life was to "raise humanity to better things." Charlotte wrote a friend that the tester told her he had "come across few girls in his 27 years of experience with as high integrity and moral standard as I."[25]

Elinor could take her bearings from Charlotte, or any of them, and know what was expected of her. That didn't mean she would do it. If she decided in favour of one of the baser emotions she could always get away with it, for she had a light heart and a genuine sense of humour and fun, and her family enjoyed this — more or less. One family friend remembered that if Marjorie and Donald got too tyrannical or stuffy Elinor would simply hide objects they needed and then spend hours "helping" to look for them. Or she would dream up other methods of "plaguing" them, like loud singing.

Impishness and fun. Curiosity. Physical vigour. Elinor's musings on her early years in Winnipeg are full of these images. She spent summers happily tearing around *Lake of the Woods* cottage country with Grace Cameron, whose parents and Elinor's rented a cottage together. Except for being forced to sit quietly for an hour after lunch and hem tea towels while being read the classics, the girls were free. One spring Elinor discovered the pile of unhemmed towels early, and she and Grace secretly and gleefully hemmed them all ahead of time. This almost undid Margaret completely, when she went to hand round the towels at the cottage. Any change in routine, however tiny, upset her terribly. "Gracie" and "Nor" did gain a few extra hours of freedom, though, for one summer anyway.

In winter, Elinor and her friends on Kennedy Street tramped a mile and a half to Kelvin High School in the morning, home for lunch, back to school and back again at day's end. Their moccasins rarely got a chance to dry fully and for months the smell of melting snow and thawing moccasins permeated the classroom. No matter how cold it got, the youngsters were never allowed to take the streetcar. But cadging rides on delivery sleighs was fair game and, in any case, the activity was unstoppable. Eaton's sleighs were best. Every morning dozens of them, red, white and blue and piled with packages, would leave the stalls and fan out across the city. The drivers were young, cheerful men who drove at a fast clip and didn't mind a few hardy souls clinging to the heavy wire netting surrounding the parcels. Empty coal wagons were another possibility. They were more comfortable, with wider runners to balance on, but the catch was having to brave the older, grouchier type of driver who tended to beat his horse and use rather shocking language.

Evenings presented more opportunities for fresh air and

exertion. Elinor spent them skating and snowshoeing on the frozen rivers or whizzing down carefully constructed ice chutes on tobaggans. Saturday afternoons, though, she was often inside the theatre watching installments of *The Perils of Pauline.* She returned each week to find out how the heroine escaped certain death from screeching trains or boiling oil.

On really special occasions there was Shakespeare at the Walker Theatre or the Minneapolis Symphony in the concert hall in the Industrial Bureau. In the same hall, Elinor once saw the famed revivalist preacher Gypsy Smith. She became so transported by his message that Charlotte had to hold her back from "prancing down to the front to be saved."[26]

The Industrial Bureau, an old barn of a building once used as a railway station, was also where Elinor went to art classes. She did this mainly to please her father. *His* father had been an art master at the Perth Academy and had exhibited in the Royal Academy. Frank himself loved sketching and doing water colours of nature scenes, and Frank thought Elinor, of his four children, had inherited something of the family talent. So she went to art school in the Bureau, passing agricultural displays of wheat and soil samples on her way upstairs to the white-walled room filled with plaster heads, torsos and grape clusters. She reproduced all these on paper, especially the busts of Dante and Voltaire, and she was good at it. Later, in medical school, when everyone had to sketch dissections, Elinor's rats appeared ready to jump off the page — in spite of being quite evidently eviscerated. But Elinor sat in front of a resistant blank page when instructed to draw something original. She said the Muse failed her.

Art school was important because it led Elinor, many years later, to an English artist named Annie French Rhead. Rhead's work hung on the walls of the school and Elinor was entranced by such tiny, intricate designs, bedecked and embellished almost beyond belief. Elinor adopted Rhead's fanciful style. This exasperated her father. *His* style, which happened to be one of broad, sweeping vistas, was not emulated by his daughter at all although he knew she was capable of it. One of the reasons he joined the Canadian Alpine Society and took her along on hill-climbing and sketching expeditions was so she would appreciate landscape. But Elinor was a willful contrary. When nudged in one direction, she always did the direct opposite. If nudged harder, she dug in her heels in prideful and stubborn defence of her choice. Where would it lead?

Charlotte may have been pondering this question when Elinor approached her to sign her "autograph book." Like many teenage girls, Elinor had such a book, the kind that's about five inches square and taken around to relatives and friends to fill with poems and rhymes, riddles and declarations of devotion. Charlotte, naturally, was the first person Elinor invited to "autograph" it. Her beloved sister penned a harsh warning entitled "Every Maid":

> King's daughter!
> Would'st thou be all fair
> Without — within,
> Peerless and beautiful,
> A very queen?
> Know then —
> Not as men build unto the Silent One,
> With clang and clamor,
> Traffic of rude voices,
> Clink of steel on stone,
> Din of hammer;
> Not so the temple of thy grace is reared.
> But — in the inmost shrine
> Must thou begin,
> And build with care,
> A Holy place,
> A place unseen;

Each stone a prayer:
And, having built,
Thy shrine sweep bare
Of self and sin
And all that might demean;
And with endeavor,
Watching ever, praying ever,
Keep it fragrant, sweet and clean.
So, by God's grace, it be fit place
His Christ shall enter and shall dwell therein.
Not as earthly fane — where chase
Of steel on stone may strive to win
Some outward grace:
Thy temple's face is chiselled from within.[27]

She signed it simply, "your sister Charlotte," and under her signature wrote a pointed question — "Do you remember the CGIT [Canadian Girls in Training] camp August 1921?" Had Elinor been showing off, or rebelling against and mocking "every maid's" role?

In choosing this poem, Charlotte consciously or unconsciously put her finger on what Elinor most needed to learn and never would — to save something, to build something inside for when the chase and the fame were over. To honour a muse. Of course, the poem is skewed too far the other way, attempting to browbeat girls into staying out of *all* spheres of action. Elinor rejected that message, understandably, but she also rejected the kernel of truth it contained. She *liked* hammers (real or symbolic) and she liked the race, rude voices and all. Clang and clamour, din and traffic, steel on stone — it was all music to her ears. She wanted to build as men did and she wanted the outward grace they got — recognition, letters after their names, prizes, money, freedom. Forget watchful maids and their temples chiselled from within where no one saw the results. She'd get around to that if and when she had time.

On the page facing Charlotte's contribution is another poem, and this one, copied in by high-school friend Effie Flanagan, is called "Achievements." It's a head-on challenge to "Every Maid," and it's easy to see its appeal for Elinor:

> Trust in thine own untried capacity
> As thou wouldst trust in God Himself,
>   Thy soul
> Is but an emanation from the whole.
> Thou dost not dream what forces lie
>   in thee,
> Vast and unfathomed as the grandest sea.
> Thy silent mind o'er diamond caves may roll.
> Go seek them — and let pilot will control
> Those passions which thy passing winds can be.
> No man shall place a limit in thy strength;
> Such triumphs as no mortal ever gained
> May yet be thine if thou wilt but
>   believe
> In thy Creator and thyself. At length
> Some feet will tread all heights now
>   unattained —
> Why not thine own? Press on;
>   Achieve! achieve.[28]

Elinor gave her whole-hearted allegiance to the tenets expressed in this sonnet — will over emotion, belief in oneself, and faith in the inevitable happy outcome of hard work and determination. She would need these qualities and more. Effie's encouragement came at a good time. In 1922, Donald was back living at home, out of uniform and in medical school. He was getting on Elinor's nerves more than ever.

What went on behind his quiet, cool exterior? Around him, all Elinor's witticisms fell flat (mainly because Donald was incapable of letting an exaggeration go uncorrected) and she got nothing but a sort of distant disapproval. It drove her crazy. Donald's reputation as a scholar bothered her too. She was good at school, but she did not do quite as well in maths as in literature and French. Her desire to be seen as smart was strong. Once she wrote to her mother, who was visiting relatives: "We had an Algebra exam the other day and I got 64. There was one question that was right that [the teacher] didn't see and another one was right or at least the same as all the other girls' and she counted it wrong. So although she may only put 64 on my report I know in my conscience & family that I got 80."[29]

Being popular and loved (adored by the Stoughtons) was not enough. Brains — "real" brains — were what counted. It was Donald who was treated so respectfully. Frank was keenly interested in his son's studies; he'd always wanted to study medicine himself but he'd had to leave home at 16 and work. Now it was as though Donald were doing it for both of them.

And not only was Donald going to medical school, the proud parents could tell the neighbours, but at the end of it he was also going to put his talents and training at the service of God. Elinor seethed. Donald — eldest, only boy, war veteran, brilliant and now . . . *medical missionary*. How, Elinor raged inwardly, was she ever going to be able to top this?

She tried to show her parents that medicine interested her as much as it did Donald. When they were away, Elinor's letters to them noted small local outbreaks of illness, and the fact a neighbour was put under chloroform to have his arm x-rayed. Elinor even diagnosed a malingerer: "Miss Wilson has been in bed to-day with what she says is a sick headache, but for dinner to-night (which she had in bed) she ate a glass dishfull of 1/2 whipped cream, 1/4 fruit & 1/4 jelly! You would have a pretty light headache to stand that!"[30]

Scores of future patients would come into contact with this "try a little starch in your backbone" attitude, already set in the young medico. But the day she would ever *have* patients must have seemed very far away. Her parents expected all their children to justify their existence by making some sort of contribution to the larger good. But virtually nobody, parents included, expected Elinor's contribution to match Donald's. How could it? She was only Babe, a beautiful girl who bubbled over with spirit and vitality. But that had value enough for most people.

Reinforcing this idea were the continuing Stoughton photo sessions. Elinor was dressed in costumes, requested to gaze raptly at some shiny *objet d'art*, posed in front of windows. She was admired, but the active role, the accomplishment, was Pater's.

The photo sessions were about to give Elinor what she later described as a "severe jolt." Donna and Pater thought it would be artistic for Elinor to take her clothes off and have some "draped" pictures taken. This suggestion embarrassed Elinor almost speechless, but she managed to convey a negative reaction to it. Well, how about just removing her middy and exposing her shoulders? No. She conceded to take off her sailor collar and hold a piece of chiffon tucked into the neckline. Not too revealing, but the incident bothered Elinor enough to tell her mother about it. Her mother agreed that nude photography was not for her daughter, regardless of artistic merit and so, Elinor wrote, "that was the end of the matter for the time being."[31]

It's highly unlikely that Elinor mentioned the incident to her father. Normal teenage embarrassment and the high level of modesty practised in what many family friends described as a "Victorian" household would have prevented her speaking. Besides, once again, her father was mostly out of the picture. In addition to his long hours at work, he was an elder at Augustine Presbyterian Church (now Augustine United), leader of bible classes at St. Andrews, chairman of the Manitoba YMCA (serving also on the national board), an executive on the Board of Trade and an executive on the board of the Canadian Club. When would she have told him? And Frank was about to get busier. His next move was into politics.

In 1922, The United Farmers of Manitoba formed the provincial government. Frank had not run in the election but was approached afterward and offered the job of treasurer and minister of Telephones. He accepted. Two northern constituencies had not yet elected candidates because of the difficulties in travelling to the regions. Frank ran in one of them, Rupert's Land, and gained a seat in the House. He started his new career in August, a few weeks before Elinor's seventeenth birthday. Donald recorded this impression of the period:

> He worked very hard during these years and they took a great deal out of him. Night after night he would return to his office to catch up on work which had been interfered with by frequent callers and other interruptions during the day. He frequently complained of being very tired and did not sleep well. Perhaps the home on Kennedy Street was really too close to his office in the Parliament [sic] Buildings and it was too easy to slip across for an extra hour or two. When he decided to enter the Government, there was some question in the minds of friends who knew him well as to whether, with his sensitive nature, he could take the rough and tumble of political debate but he stood up well.[32]

The pressure was intense, and when the House wasn't sitting Frank took month-long business trips and made visits to the distant riding he represented. When the House was in session, Elinor, who lived directly across from the Legislature, could slip into the Visitor's Gallery and watch her father. He was once named the best dressed man in the House and always wore the conventional white piping along the lapels of his vest. With his height and dignified bearing, high forehead and pince-nez glasses, he looked the very picture of impeccable Presbyterian solidity. He acted it too. It was Frank who moved in the House that Members' indemnities be cut from $1,800 to $1,500 to set a good example to others and to counter what he called the drift toward over-spending.[33]

The 1924 session was full of problems. Donald relates in his biography that some people, including Frank, felt the lieutenant-governor, Sir J.A.M. Aikins, was trying to exert undue influence. Aikins was demanding that copies of all bills to come before the House should be submitted to him in advance and he insisted on changes to many of them. He used the pressure tactic of delaying approval on money bills that had already been passed. Here was a matter of principle *par excellence* for Frank, and he was not likely to miss it. While the premier and the attorney general were less inclined to force a confrontation, Frank insisted that it was a vital constitutional matter. He resigned. Elinor later quoted him as saying that "a man could not be a Christian and a politician."[34]

Things were in something of an upheaval in Frank's *other* house too — the one on Kennedy Street. Donald had gradu-ated from medical college — an alumni medalist and winner of the Chown prize in surgery — and was getting married and sailing to Formosa to take up his mission duties. The Blacks were hosting the reception at their house, and Margaret was planning this in meticulous detail.

In addition to that stress, it wasn't a particularly happy or united family at the moment. Elinor had recently started medical school. It's reasonable to suppose that Charlotte supported her sister (given the fact she later helped Elinor financially), but Frank, Margaret and especially Donald re-mained sturdily opposed. Donald knew that women were barely tolerated in the medical faculty. And Elinor would have to study and expose herself to material he felt wasn't proper for a woman to see. Furthermore, in his opinion, women didn't have the physical strength for some aspects of the profession. Overall, he told Elinor coldly, *women were nothing but a nuisance in medical schools.*

Elinor had ignored the pall of disapproval and gone ahead ("she was just bent on doing it," one relative recalled). But she was bitterly hurt and disappointed, especially in her brother. In spite of her mischief and mixed feelings, she'd tried hard to win his approval. Now she resolved to distance herself as much as possible. Elinor joined the basketball team, she said later, "so people would know I was different from Donald." She told others that Donald was the scholar and she was the athlete. She went so far as to compete in basketball meets when she had her period. Margaret was shocked. She even wrote to Donald to enlist his help in stopping such a risky, not to mention immodest, practice. She also took one of Elinor's dates aside at the door and asked him if he thought Elinor's athletics and athletic shorts were proper.

Elinor didn't care what any of them thought. She proudly donned the skull-and-crossbones uniform and went out for track and field as well. She became an inter-varsity champion shotputter and high jumper. And, as she flew over the barriers on the track, looking, as her yearbook put it, like "a Greek goddess,"[35] Donald's remark echoed until it took on a life of its own. She vowed to do well, so well that one day she could take those stinging words — and fling them back in his face.

▼ Two▼

REBELLION
AND ESCAPE
▼

*It was under the influence of this optimism that young
women cherished ambitions for the wider exercise of their
individual powers, and saw no limit to the kind and
quality of service which they might offer to the
community. (Winifred Holtby, on post-war optimism and
1920s' womanhood.)*

ELINOR'S OUTRAGE, especially at her brother, was part of
something larger than family dynamics. It was 1925, she was
20, and it was the New Day. Optimism and opportunity
seemed infinite, cooperation and reason were bound to triumph, and it was idealistic youth, Elinor and her friends, who
were going to make sure of it. Winifred Holtby, one of Elinor's
favourite writers, looked back on this time and wrote, "Old
hampering conventions had broken down; superstitions were
destroyed; the young had come into their kingdom."[1] Elinor
must have felt this was true everywhere but in *her* family.

"The upbringing in the [Black] home was *so* strict," said
one friend of the family, "not a word out of place." She

remembered Elinor coming over to her house to read "the funny papers." Comics weren't allowed at the Blacks'. Another friend recalled always feeling that Elinor's parents were so *old*, even though, upon reflection, she realized they were the same age as her own parents. Small wonder Elinor was feeling stifled, rebellious — and resentful that Donald was siding with the old order.

But her brother's opposition was understandable, if not admirable. Donald was 29, not 20, and his major choices — a traditional wife and the mission field — were behind him. Furthermore, he too was part of a bigger picture, namely the long, miserable story of men versus women in medicine.

Consider, for example, the manifesto issued by the Philadelphia County Medical Society in 1867. It suggested that the "physiological peculiarities of women, even in single life, and the disorders consequent on them, cannot fail, frequently, to interfere with the regular discharge of her duties as physician. . . . The delicate organization and predominance of the nervous system render her peculiarly susceptible to suffer, if not to sink, under the fatigue and mental shocks which she must encounter in her professional round. Man, with his robust frame and trained self-command, is often barely equal to the task."[2]

Women probably found this assertion as ludicrous in 1867 as they would now — but what followed was serious. Male medical students spat tobacco juice at the women who tried to attend lectures and intimidated them by jeering and cursing.

A few years later, Dr. Edward Clarke published theories somewhat similar to those in the Philadelphia manifesto, but he had a much wider influence. His premise was that girls simply could not, without serious damage, divert the flow of blood from building "a large and complicated reproductive mechanism" to the brain. They shouldn't be expected to, he argued. He admitted the girls he studied *seemed* able to combine school and adolescence, they *appeared* to actually thrive on learning, but the end result of mixing education and ovary-building was inevitably hysteria, dysmenorrhea, invalidism, insanity and even death. He provided a selection of gruesome case histories as proof, including the story of Miss D.

> Miss D—— went to college in good physical condition. During the four years of her college life, her parents and college faculty required her to get what is popularly called an education. Nature required her, during the same period, to build and put in working-order a large and complicated reproductive mechanism. . . . She naturally obeyed the requirements of the faculty, which she could see, rather than the requirements of the mechanism within her, which she could not see. . . . The stream of vital and constructive force evolved within her was turned steadily to the brain, and away from the ovaries and their accessories. The result of this sort of education was, that these last-mentioned organs, deprived of sufficient opportunity and nutriment, first began to perform their functions with pain, a warning of error that was unheeded; then, to cease to grow; next, to set up once a month a grumbling torture that made life miserable; and lastly, the brain and the whole nervous system, disturbed, in obedience to the law, that, if one member suffers, all the members suffer, became neuralgic and hysterical.[3]

Miss D. somehow escaped being "consigned to an asylum" but many of Dr. Clarke's other patients did not. He called the image of an American girl, "yoked" with a dictionary, "an exhibition of monstrous brain and aborted ovarian development."[4] His book, *Sex in Education; Or, A Fair Chance for the Girls*, was so popular it went through several editions, the second a week after the first.

Some bad ideas stay around a long time. One of Donald's main arguments, 50 years later, was that women were too delicate to be doctors: they didn't have what it took; they couldn't stand the pace.

Women entered medical school in Canada in 1881. At first, the three female medical students admitted to Queen's University in Kingston, Ontario, were treated well. If an "awkward" subject was discussed (like obstetrics), they sat in a little room adjacent to the classroom, thereby saving everyone from embarrassment.[5]

However, the second year was more difficult. One of the women wrote in her diary, "No-one knows or can know what a furnace we are passing through these days at the College. We suffer torment, we shrink inwardly, we are hurt cruelly."[6] Carlotta Hacker, in her book, *The Indomitable Lady Doctors*, tells the story of how, after a progressive and influential group of seniors graduated, the women found themselves at the mercy of classmates who were bent on making their lives miserable, egged on by the lecturer in physiology.[7]

It got rougher. One might even say ruthless. The people of Kingston generally supported the women, so to sway public opinion to their side the male students claimed that lectures were being glossed over or not taught in sufficient detail because it was necessary to consider the women's modesty. The men weren't getting their money's worth. Ultimatum — *get rid of the women or we'll move, en masse, to Trinity College in Toronto.* Trinity agreed to take the men. Neither Queen's nor the town of Kingston could survive an economic blow like that. A compromise was reached — the three women could finish out their course, taking *all* their classes separately from the men. No new women would be admitted.[8]

The tactics used at Queen's in 1882 are interesting. It wasn't suggested that the women couldn't handle the work. It was just that, with these little adjacent rooms and garbled lectures and upset faculty, they got in the way. *They were nothing but a nuisance.*

Elinor's own training ground, the University of Manitoba

Medical College, presented yet another aspect of the challenge women took on to become doctors. The message was not "we don't think you can do it" or "we won't let you try." It was more "come if you must but you'd better blend in." That meant, for women, checking half their identity at the door. As a close woman friend of Elinor's, also a doctor, put it, "Women were women and men were men. And doctors were men."

In fact, there were female physicians in Manitoba before there was a medical college. And from the first few who arrived — Dr. Charlotte Ross and Drs. Amelia and Lillian Yeoman (mother and daughter) — there has been an unbroken line of women doctors in the province. But the story of the founding of the Medical College, and the language used to tell the story, illustrate just how masculine a profession medicine was perceived to be.

The Manitoba Medical College got its start in 1883 when a group of enterprising would-be students learned that a Toronto doctor was trying to make a deal with the premier to open a "proprietary" medical school. (These money-making operations, widespread until 1910, had short medical courses, low academic standards and high profit margins.) The group knew that local doctors had moved, successfully, to place a prior claim that would affiliate the future college with the University of Manitoba where it would be run properly. The group also knew that the main objective of these Winnipeg doctors was really to shut out the man from Toronto, not to run a school, and the doctors now planned to drop the whole thing for a few years. After all, there was no money for teachers or buildings.

The would-be students thought otherwise. They boldly ran a notice in the Free Press calling a meeting of all medical students for the purpose of establishing a course of lectures. They were opposed, of course, by the conservative-minded, but they won. In less than a month, the first set of lectures was taking place.

This is an exploit worth celebrating and at least two college histories have done so. One of them describes these early teachers and students as having "the stuff that draws men of character to the turbulence and rigors of the frontier."[9] Another article calls them "frontiersmen, hard working, hard living general practitioners all; strange acolytes yet true Aesculapians, sons of Hippocrates." The story of these men is "a story to stir the blood" and the first dean of medicine was the "dean of the brotherhood."[10]

This was the tactic that would touch Elinor the deepest and the longest. Invisibility. How could Elinor, or any young woman, reading this, hearing this language, see herself as one of them, as a doctor? Where did she fit in this picture? Well, that was her problem. Elinor wouldn't be hearing too much about "sons and daughters of Hippocrates." Once she picked up a stethoscope, it was going to be "the brotherhood" the whole way, including "Fellows" of the Royal College and letters addressed to dear sir. She could take it or leave it. If she chose to take it, she'd better learn to take it like a man.

Donald knew this. When he was going through in 1921 there were 8,706 doctors in Canada; 98.3 percent of them were men.[11] All Donald had to do was look around him to see what the odds were of Elinor retaining any vestige of the feminine qualities he and his parents had, heaven knew, tried to instill in her. No, he couldn't support her choice.

And if Elinor could have looked ahead 30 years, she might have had second thoughts herself. But in 1925, she had no doubts; 1925 was what Elinor had on her side against all the arguments and all the statistics. Timing. It was luckier even than having her next set of patrons waiting in the wings. Elinor had a brave new world and the economy backing her up.

In Manitoba, crops were "abundant to phenomenal" and prices were high. In Winnipeg, luxury furs were selling fast.[12] So were crystal radios, and people were thrilled to inform each other, "I got Minneapolis!"[13] The mayor of Winnipeg was happily planning a flamboyant "Pine to Palm" motorcade of Winnipeggers driving to New Orleans to promote their city to American tourists. The Winnipeg Grain Exchange was building the largest office building in Canada. The Hudson's Bay Company launched construction of a department store covering an entire city block and intended to rival any store in New York.[14] The Winnipeg history, *An Apple for the Teacher*, summed it all up this way: "1925: Good times continuing; Jeremiahs laughed at."[15] With everything going so well, society could afford to be generous to women.

Good times gave Elinor a boost over that first barrier of family opposition. Good times helped her into medical school. It was hard work that ensured she stayed there. Hard work, and the inspiration of an extraordinary role model named Gertrude.

Gertrude Rutherford was not a doctor. But the world she manoeuvred in so successfully was just as masculine and rigidly hierarchical as medicine. Her sphere was the church, and more specifically, the Student Christian Movement (SCM). Gertrude was a driving force behind this interesting and radical social movement; when she toured nationally to meet and encourage SCM groups on campus, people knew they were in the company of a Presence.

Gertrude was a big, tall woman, one of the few women who could look Elinor right in the eye. She moved in national and international circles in such a way that men and women deferred to her large spirit and larger vision. One friend of Gertrude's wrote Elinor, "It's wonderful to see keen minds in action and to hear men talk as those men did. G.L.R. was the only woman who could hold her own with them."[16] Elinor called Gertrude Prince. Other women just called her Boss.

Gertrude had a mission — to open the church to women. After Church Union in 1925, Gertrude worked for the United Church, an institution that did not ordain a woman minister until 1939. Gertrude saw the church as a place where women could make a vital contribution, not as volunteers or help-meets, but as professional administrators. She promoted this career option to young women and she worked tirelessly behind the scenes to create the environment she envisaged.

For several years, Gertrude's vision dovetailed with what was happening in the SCM. She liked being around students and young people, and some of the brightest minds were drawn to this movement, which encouraged them — almost forced them — to question, question, question.

Anyone could join the movement. It wasn't necessary to believe in Christianity; it *was* a requirement to be willing to test one's beliefs. No one could parrot what he or she had been taught or had always assumed to be true. Members had to study "The Records"[17] directly and ask questions. Stretching their minds and ideas, students struggled with the questions under the direction of national leaders like movement founder Dr. Henry Sharman, Gertrude, and Murray Brooks. They gathered at Camp Minnising in Algonquin Park or Jasper Park in Alberta and they worked hard. One woman recalled it as far more rigorous than any university course she took.

Dr. Sharman believed it his duty to "disturb complacent and unquestioning acceptance, and to compel students to arrive at conclusions which they could sustain."[18] Naturally, in such an atmosphere, everything was eventually called into question — the war, institutions like the YMCA and the church, parental values, the divinity of Jesus, relationships between men and women — everything. There were partici-

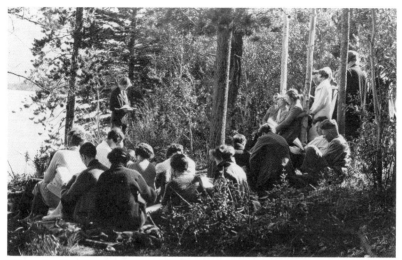

Elinor leading morning worship at SCM camp gathering,
Jasper, July 1928

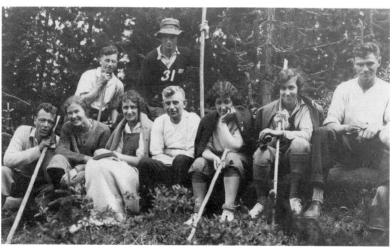

Elinor, second from right, at SCM camp, Jasper, July 1928

pants who found the experience liberating, for others it was frightening. For some, it left an "indelible imprint."

Elinor went to these conferences, and for one year she was SCM president at the university and led the weekly study sessions. There's no evidence that it left a dramatic imprint on her, except in terms of the people she met and stayed friends with the rest of her life. She enjoyed the camping and the intellectual challenge but soul-searching was not really her style. The SCM *was* a way to keep in touch with Gertrude, though, and that relationship was something that did affect her.

Aside from the fact that there were no such female role-models around the medical department, Gertrude was special. She was supremely capable, combining vision with practical help. When she found an eager young woman with potential, she acted. One such woman wrote this about Gertrude's influence on her life, emphasizing that her story was typical:

> It was she who made sure I got to Dr. Sharman's study Seminar at Minnising the summer before I became local SCM secretary at Alberta. And she again who urged me to go to Europe the summer before I became a Nat'l SCM secretary (1934) in Toronto; who loaned me the $400 I needed to get there & back, & arranged for me to share a cabin with a young prof. of French at Victoria College; she who wrote to people to look out for me at the International Conferences I was to attend. . . . She continued to open doors for me after I started my job — and hers was always open. . . . When I had to have surgery, it was Gertrude who arranged that her sister Louella be my "special" nurse; & Gertrude again who persuaded her cousin . . . that I'd be an excellent chauffeur-companion to accompany her on her winter trip to Bahamas — at a time when I was in need of a convalescent holiday.[19]

Elinor never detailed Gertrude's help to her in this way. She simply said, when she was at the height of her career,

"Had it not been for her, I certainly would not be heading a Dept today — & that's the truth I'm telling you!"[20] With younger women, Gertrude was described as tough in her questioning and her expectations, but at the same time "she was confident that you could do it."[21] Gertrude had faith in women as professionals and shapers of policy, and, for Elinor, that was a refreshing change from the home front. Gertrude could pass on the benefit of her years of experience as a career woman. Through example, if nothing else, she helped Elinor stay the course.

And what a course it was. Fortunately, Elinor's father accepted a job offer in Kelowna in 1927 and that gave her some badly needed breathing space to concentrate on her work. She and her parents were *not* getting along. Elinor could hold a grudge at least as well as anyone else in the family, and she was not going to forgive Margaret and Frank for their failure to understand her ambition. They responded with endless sermons.

Before leaving Winnipeg, her parents installed Elinor in a boarding house that cost $32 a month. Her monthly allowance from Frank for all her expenses was $40. As Elinor wryly noted in the Stoughton memoir, she was free, but she wasn't exactly in a position to go wild. The ever-present Stoughtons were delighted to make life less austere. They provided exotic meals in their elegant apartment, gave her silk pajamas, and naturally invited "Sweet Childe" along on any cultural outings. They may have deplored Elinor's habit of entering a room "as if she were going to a fire," but, deportment aside, Elinor could bask in uncritical adoration. None of this made going home any easier.

Her first visit to Kelowna was a disaster. There was one opportunity for some comic relief but it was missed. Frank had bought his first car — a 1927 Buick Coach with a fabric top and demountable rims. He and Elinor taught themselves to drive it, using trial and error, and both of them were bribing the mechanic to take small dents out of the car before the other one could notice. A good laugh over this might have broken the impasse. But the mechanic kept his word, and Elinor and her father couldn't share the joke — they were barely speaking. When she returned to Winnipeg, her mother sent her this rebuke:

> In some ways you disappointed very greatly this summer, Elinor. . . . You were constantly impatient with Daddy — at times really insolent — careless in your speech and adopting more and more ugly slang expressions in spite of my protests. Now Elinor, if a mother ever loved a daughter — you know that I have loved you and have been proud of you. I do not want you to be a prim prig — but a girl living up to the privilege of culture which has been yours — unselfish enough to overlook failings — faults perhaps — in those who have willingly, gladly made sacrifices for you — and continue to do so. . . . No one can be more bright and interesting than you — *when you feel like* — that is one great reason why your indifference *hurts.* . . .
>
> What I want to convey to you is my longing for you to be a girl of refinement and with ideals above the common underprivileged sort — avoid coarseness in speech and action — this has crept into your manner. . . . You must be ever watchful — more than most people you absorb the speech and manners of those you associate with and like.[22]

Margaret was right on this last point. Elinor was an excellent mimic and could blend into a milieu expertly. And of course, as she was surrounded almost exclusively by male students and teachers, theirs were the mannerisms she absorbed. Just the "coarsening" effect Margaret and Donald had feared, but for Elinor, it was a survival mechanism that worked beautifully. She was as popular as ever. She passed second year with honours, and aced physical diagnosis.

In third year, the work became even more absorbing. With much of the laboratory work behind her, she could concentrate on the fascinating world of human beings and everything that went wrong with them. And in fourth year, there were the maternity calls.

The fourth-year class was divided into groups of 12 or 14 and each group had to observe 25 births. Group division was done as much as possible by geography because of the night calls. In the daytime, it was easy to assemble the group. Everyone was either at a lecture, a clinic or an autopsy. But at night, one student was designated the caller. The hospital called him or her, and the caller called all the others, and finally a cab. None of this was much appreciated by Elinor's landlady.

But Elinor loved squeezing into the cab in dead of night, waking up on the way, scrambling into a gown and mask and taking her place on the two-step platform "at the business end of the table." Lowly students were excluded from going to the West 4 kitchen for the "fourth stage of labour"; that was where the obstetrician, residents and interns went after the case was concluded. Everyone made toast and drank coffee, and interns got a chance to ask the questions that might have shown them up in front of students.

By Elinor's own intern year she was out of the boarding house and virtually living at the hospital. Male interns *were* living there, but since there were no quarters for women the hospital rented a nearby apartment for them. Elinor and the two other women interns shared the apartment and took their meals in the nurses' residence.

This segregation made it easier for one of the teachers to call an impromptu clinic at a highly unusual time — Sunday morning. The topic was birth control. It was illegal for doctors to provide it or even advise it, so birth control was not exactly on the official curriculum. Nonetheless, what little there was to tell was passed on in this special clinic. But not to the three women. They weren't invited.

Even if the women had known about it, they may not have found the time or energy to lobby for inclusion. It was such a hectic period. On top of all their other responsibilities, interns did their own lab work — urinalyses, blood counts, grouping and matching blood. There was no blood bank.

When a patient needed a transfusion, doctors turned to a list of donors (usually medical students who needed the money). Sometimes the patient's relatives were called in. When a match was found, the patient (on the operating table) and the donor (on a stretcher) lay head to foot. One doctor took a 50-cc syringe and inserted it into the donor's arm. When the syringe was full it was handed to another doctor to inject into the patient. The process seemed agonizingly slow.

The rotation through anaesthesia was even more harrowing. Interns reeked of ether for two months. Nothing would take the smell off. But that was the least of it. The real problem was the lack of training or supervision. One doctor described it this way: "If you were a doctor you could give an anaesthetic. And we were sent [alone], in our very first days as an intern, to the operating room to give anaesthetics. Isn't that horrible?"[23]

Elinor thought so. She hated the procedure. Most anaesthetics were a mixture of ether and chloroform. The solution was dribbled on a mask made of several layers of gauze, saturating an area not larger than a nickel. The intern had to watch the eyes (to determine what stage the patient had reached) and the mask. A too-wet mask could cause burns to the patient's face. With certain anaesthetics, patients went through a brief restless or even obstreperous stage before sedation. Elinor misjudged a dose once and the patient jumped right off the table. This happened to others too. But worst of all were patients who held their breath and then gulped for air. If the air was too saturated with chloroform, the heart stopped. (Maternal mortality statistics for 1927 for the Winnipeg General Hospital reported 53 deaths — eight from asphyxiation or chloroform narcosis.[24])

It was a relief for Elinor to finish the rotation and go on to internal medicine. There, one of Elinor's teachers had a stethoscope with eight rubber tubes. Up to eight students got to listen to a patient's heart at the same time. That was mildly amusing and it didn't kill anyone.

But the specialty that caught and held Elinor's attention was obstetrics and gynaecology. She had a practical and mechanical turn of mind. To her, the art of obstetrics was rather like carpentry: one had to understand precise angles, and be good with tools and one's hands. And at the end of it one had something to show for it. All that was appealing. Then there was the gynaecology side, the only opportunity to do surgery a woman doctor was likely to get. Finally, Elinor thought the teachers in ob-gyne were special. She wrote a history of the department 50 years after she first met them, but she recalled those men vividly.[25]

There was Dr. Olafur Bjornson — a flat-faced man who put Elinor in mind of a large, comforting rag doll wearing glasses. First impressions can be misleading. "O.B." had a biting wit and was standing by, "making his usual derisive remarks" the day Elinor had her first forceps case.[26] It was a nerve-wracking experience.

O.B. expected every pregnancy to be completely normal, so he paid little attention to pre-natal care and he hated episiotomies. Even forceps were seldom used. His patients were always delivered lying on their sides. Elinor didn't always agree with his methods; she thought they exhausted the mothers and put some babies at risk. But she credited O.B. with teaching her manual dexterity.

Dr. Frederick Gallagher McGuinness was just the opposite. His patients were delivered lying on their backs. Elinor described him as "an enthusiastic user of episiotomy" whose cases "did not take nearly as long to deliver as did O.B.'s."[27] He repaired the episiotomies with three through-and-through sutures. Elinor used to wince, watching. She knew the healing would be slow and painful.

Elinor described McGuinness as tall and handsome; she once called him "a fine broth of a lad." She also recognized him as a very good teacher who happily announced "like so!" whenever he demonstrated the movements that could prevent a breech birth. Nonetheless, she didn't like him, and this enmity grew.

She adored Dr. Daniel Sayre MacKay. He was short and stocky, and had served with the Queen's Own Cameron Highlanders in The Great War. He retained his military bearing, parade-ground voice and strict adherence to form, but his attempts at being a real martinet were doomed to failure. Elinor described him as "incurably tender hearted." He gave lavish Sunday dinner parties for impoverished interns. He taught gynaecology, not obstetrics, and Elinor thought he was an excellent surgeon — with a few strange "foibles."

The most visible MacKay quirk was the apron. No matter how hot it was outside (and his operating room always had to be at least 80 degrees to start with), Dr. MacKay wore a pink rubber apron that covered him from head to foot and wrapped well around the back. He never perspired; the students and patients were sopping.

He didn't want his view of an operation obstructed by assistants wielding sponges, so he arranged for a steady stream of sterile water over the area instead. The theatre was soon awash, with everyone's feet soaking wet. None of his patients were allowed to sit up for 10 days after an operation, and for the first 24 hours they could be given nothing but ice chips.

All this was nothing compared to his treatments for

gynaecological disorders. He believed that an "ovarian tubercle" in the nostril became congested at the time of menstruation, caused nosebleeds and reduced heavy menstrual flow. Dysmenorrhea (painful periods) could be relieved by using an extract from the mammary glands called "mammose." An injection of boiled milk into the buttock of a woman suffering from pelvic inflammatory disease was beneficial because it caused a high temperature.[28]

It's obvious the experience of accompanying "D.S." on public rounds was not to be missed. He led his retinue of students, nurses and interns around the 20-bed ward, chatting with each patient and making interesting remarks on every case. Elevators and rooms were entered and exited according to strict rules of hospital rank, people peeling off from the group like crisp bills. Everyone who could, retreated afterward to the nursing office to listen to yet more comments and stories.

MacKay was a strange choice as mentor, but that's the role he played for Elinor. He became increasingly important to her; privately he sometimes worried about pushing her too hard.

Dr. John Douglas McQueen was the man Elinor meant when she told a friend, "I can't do [your mother's] operation. It would be just like operating on my own mother. But I'll get her the best."[29] Elinor felt McQueen excelled equally in obstetrics and gynaecology.

There was some rivalry between McQueen and McGuinness, and those under them often tended toward one or the other camp. Elinor was squarely in the McQueen camp. She described him as "greatly loved and respected," also reserved, "as befitted his Scottish ancestry," and given to showing displeasure by quietly getting up and leaving. Younger colleagues worked up to calling him "J.D." — and it took them years to do it.

Elinor admired what she called his "uncanny" diagnostic skills. His technique was straightforward; examine the patient, sit and think, re-examine, resume a thoughtful silence, and finally give his opinion — "which was very rarely wrong."[30]

Dr. Rosslyn Brough Mitchell was the fifth and last man Elinor profiled in her history of the department. Like McQueen, Elinor described him as extremely kind and helpful to young doctors just starting out. He would pretend to need their advice and then slip them a five-dollar bill for the "consultation." He and McQueen set up Manitoba's first pre-natal clinic in 1921. He kept his maternity fees so low for years that other obstetricians held meetings about it. Elinor didn't list a nickname for him, as she did for the others. To her, he was Dr. Ross Mitchell, and "the dean of obstetrics in Western Canada."[31]

.These were the men who influenced, helped or obstructed Elinor for years: the obstetricians at Winnipeg General.

Elinor decided to follow in their footsteps and become one of them. But a few months before her graduation, the market crashed. Frank lost heavily. D.S. (Dr. MacKay) was hit hard by losses; rumour had it that only a fund set up by anonymous friends kept him going. Arthur Stoughton's major project — a 16-storey office tower — was stalled indefinitely. Elinor pinned her hopes for post-graduate training on an advertised junior residency in obstetrics and gynaecology at Johns Hopkins Hospital in Baltimore. She didn't get it. It looked like she was stopped before she'd even got started.

Enter Uncle Ivor and Aunt Jeannie. Jeannie was Frank Black's younger but not particularly beloved sister, and her husband Ivor was a wealthy lawyer. When Elinor heard they were coming for a visit, her depression over the Johns Hopkins set-back evaporated. Recalling her mother's words that no one could be brighter or more interesting than she

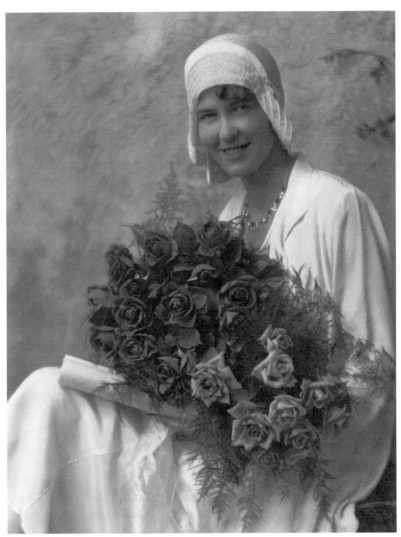

Elinor F.E. Black, M.D., May 14, 1930

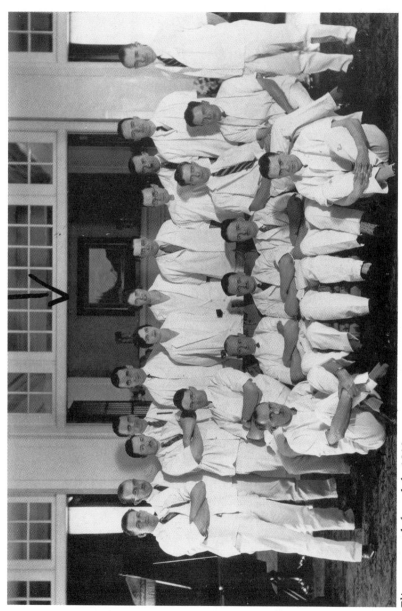

Elinor, seventh from left, 1930

could — when she felt like it — Elinor made every effort to feel like it around Jeannie and Ivor. Sure enough, shortly after their return to England, Elinor got a letter from them. In one account, Elinor reported only that the letter contained the enormous sum of $300 and expressed a desire to give her a year's post-graduate training in London. In fact, Jeannie's letter shows she wanted a playmate — and she was prepared to promise Elinor the moon to get one:

> Destroy this letter after you have *digested* the contents!!
> Dearest Elinor,
>   . . . We do so much want you over and I promise you it would be *the* year of your young life! We'd have a nice place for you to live in — in London. . . . My Dear — you'd have a ripping time. As *every* night would not be spent in study and I cd have lots of weekends in London with you. We also might sandwich in a week in Paris — and if we have you during the summer — just before you return home we'd take you on a cruise in the Mediterranean and show you Venice, Naples, Constantinople; . . . and besides all this, you'd gain so much more knowledge and experience in Medicine & Surgery. . . . We'd put certain sums in a bank in London for you and you'd have your own cheques to write and so not be dependent on asking for money; . . . so you see Dear — we are trying to give you a chance & happiness.[32]

Aunt Jeannie took parting shots at Margaret's "primness and persnickettyness" and Frank's tendency to "come to heel" before reminding Elinor that she was a "full blown medico" and of age. "So," she wrote, "don't hesitate to throw your cap over the windmill if necessary!" Not that Elinor needed much encouragement. But Jeannie suspected that Frank and Margaret would oppose the whole plan. She was right.

Besides their hurt pride at not being able to afford Elinor's education themselves, Elinor's parents thought Jeannie was unstable, given to passing whims and likely to abandon their daughter when she got tired of her. Elinor didn't want to hear about it. Luck was in the air. In addition to causing the appearance of Jeannie-genie, the summer of 1930 brought to Winnipeg the joint meeting of the British Medical Association and the Canadian Medical Association. At the meeting, Elinor managed to chat with Dame Louise McIlroy of the Royal Free Hospital in London. And that had led to an invitation to visit the august doctor when she got to England. There was no stopping Elinor now.

There *was* a three-month residency at the Children's Hospital to be done first, though. As much as her head was spinning with Jeannie's enticements, Elinor must have been diverted, at least briefly, by a new hospital environment. To start with, there was the daily entertainment provided by the hospital elevator. Because it was made of open grillwork, moved extremely slowly and was encircled by a stairway, many long conversations took place between those going up in the elevator and those climbing the stairs.[33] Whichever way Elinor got to the ward, once there she was presented with "apple-pie beds and other tomfooleries" that the young nurses had dreamed up to tease her.

There were serious moments too. She saw compassion and the class system at work when doctors falsely listed public patients (children whose parents couldn't pay) as dangerously ill so parents could visit more often. Normally, public patients could have visitors only on Wednesdays and Sundays, from 2:00 p.m to 3:30. Paying patients could have visitors every day.[34]

It was absorbing, it was more experience, but she knew paediatrics was not her niche and London was never far from her thoughts. From the hospital, she wrote to her parents:

August 17, 1930
Dear Father & Mother,
    Two months from today I land in Liverpool!! . . . For once, Father, you have mistaken Jean's judgement as she has done far more for me

towards setting me on the path to finding the course I want than I could ever have done myself.[35]

Elinor had just received another letter from Jeannie, this one describing how to behave on board the ship. Jeannie sent a thorough list of whom to tip ("Table Steward — 5 dollars or 1 pound note — *no more* — *less* if you like, Cabin Steward, Lounge Steward, Lift Boy, Boots [you may never see him], Band, Crew"), and she told Elinor to keep all passenger lists for her inspection.[36] Did any warning bells go off that this type of detailed advice seemed awfully familiar?

Elinor went to Kelowna to say goodbye; it went badly. Jeannie and Frank were warring over particulars now. Elinor's next letter from Jeannie read, "Your father had evidently written and said go from Liverpool to Joppa — but that is *all wrong*. You come home with *me* for the weekend. . . . At Joppa there is no maid, as you know — & a good deal of discomfort — the wallpapers curse at one, & the furniture also!"[37] Elinor didn't need any more discomfort than she was already facing. The atmosphere was grim and the faces long; she was desperate to be gone.

Frank's pride made him give her a letter of credit he couldn't really afford. Elinor knew better than to use it unless she were at death's door. Her own pride was at stake, and so was her independence and her belief in her decision. After a stiff farewell, she returned to Winnipeg to take the boat train to Montreal.

Donna and Pater came to the train station to see her off. They were enthusiastic about her plans and told her to write to them any time for funds. At the last minute, Donna handed her a letter. Elinor boarded, got herself settled and glanced out the window. Nothing but familiar prairie and the view wouldn't change for hours and hours. She reached for the letter.

Elinor, Sweet,

Mrs. Veitch is sticking a basketful of damson plums full of holes with a darning needle in the kitchen — with the door open between us. The sociability *per se* is delightful but it may militate against the concentration required for a letter such as this.

A railway station parting is a very unsatisfactory goodbye. When you are in the quiet of your train section or your steamer berth it will be a much better time for us to commune with each other. I hope you will open your mind and heart wide to all the enjoyment this trip is going to afford. There will be lots of nice people to meet, plenty new interesting things to do and several problems to confront. Take all these things as a great adventure and don't be afraid of man or institution or new custom. . . .

I am so glad the opportunity came to you. You have our warmest love and our best wishes, Dear Childe, for your comfort, your success, and your happiness.[38]

Well, that was more like it! Cheered by this show of support, Elinor let her dreams, held in so tightly since Kelowna, go free. She pulled out her passport and opened it, gloating. She read it all. Miss Elinor Frances Elizabeth Black, M.D. National Status: British Subject. Profession: Medical. Face: Oval. Colour of eyes: Grey. Her face looked back at her from the photo planted squarely below "Photograph of Bearer." The square next to her face was blank; it was for the photograph of the bearer's wife. One passport per family.

Elinor didn't know exactly where she was headed, but she was not likely to end up any time soon on a square marked "Wife" on some man's passport. When the train pulled into Montreal she was eager to keep moving. On to the next means of conveyance! The *Duchess of York* was a splendid name for a ship, even if more world-weary travellers called her The Drunken Duchess. They weren't going to spoil Elinor's fun.

It was a beautiful fall day as they sailed down the St. Lawrence. There was more than one kind of hurricane just ahead, but Elinor, exultant, saw nothing but blue skies and a limitless horizon.

Three

WHIRLWIND

▼

*I thought very seriously about marrying him.
(Elinor Black)*

*For a girl, getting married practically means dropping your
profession, doesn't it? (Bernard Collings)*

Going down the St. Lawrence
Duchess of York
Oct. 10/30

Dear Mother & Father —
Here I am going down the St. Lawrence at last. . . . How are you
both? Do take housework & office work less seriously this winter &
enjoy life & your wee house.

So far my trip has been thoroughly enjoyable. . . . Montreal is
quite a place — especially when it comes to the traffic. I hope the
London traffic is not much more scarey!

My cabin is a nice outside one. . . . Fortunately I am at the Chief
Engineer's table with Mrs. Russell (my train acquaintance) & some
very nice business gentlemen — not of the commercial traveller
type.

Have several other letters to catch the mail at Quebec, so I shall stop this. I hope you both have a happy & healthy winter with not too many cares.

Please don't worry about me — because I shall be OK. Au revoir. Much love — Elinor.[1]

But Frank did worry. He sent Elinor a list of codes made up of seven letters each. The codes were to be used when sending telegrams; the idea was that Elinor could explain any sort of emergency or situation in some detail while sending the most economical telegram possible. He also sent warnings about the "treachery or misery of the English climate" and the "very marked degree of indifference" to religious matters in England. He himself, he went on, was disposed, on general principle, "to suspect people who will *not* attend or interest themselves in Church effort."

He worried as well about Elinor's dangerously run-down condition — as evidenced by her negativity in Kelowna. He reminded Elinor that no one could accuse Donald of being negative. He told Elinor that she puzzled her mother, who was not well and was manifesting this in "a passionate attachment to trivial details of house-keeping — so trivial as to be exceedingly irritating to others." He ended all this with the cheerful thought — "Accident or evil would break Mother's heart. We trust you may be protected from both."[2]

Elinor's response was to stick to chatty, neutral remarks such as, "The boat itself is beautiful. The panelling is . . . most effective. Wood trimmed with contrasting wood." She did tell her father that she didn't ever want to hear him criticizing "the drunkenness of modern youth" again, after what she'd seen of the behaviour of some middle-aged commercial traveller types. But she mainly concentrated on safe topics like meals ("I have managed my three squares daily, & have wasted nothing") and weather.

Given the weather she had, Elinor's ability to eat those three squares *was* noteworthy. She wrote Frank that it was

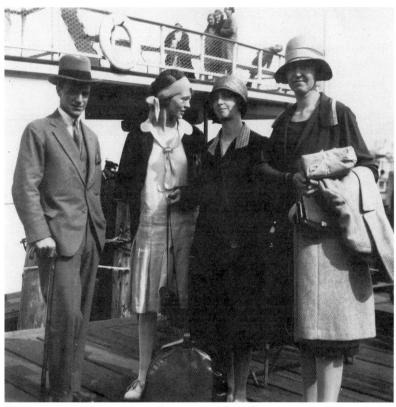

Uncle Ivor, Charlotte, Aunt Jeannie and friend

the roughest crossing the *Duchess of York* ever had, according to the "old salts" on board. The ship went "from the swell into a ninety-mile hurricane" causing, among other problems, the grand piano in the lounge to break loose and crash around wildly, scaring the blind passenger on board half to death.[3]

So it was a slightly sea-tossed young woman Aunt Jeannie bundled into a train and whisked off to her home in the village of Hessle — where Elinor discovered that she hadn't got very far from Kelowna after all. Jeannie insisted on continually advising her when to have a bath, when to change her stockings and how to part her hair.

Furthermore, Jeannie was odd. She wore a hat in her own home for lunch. Driving with her was terrifying. She appeared to have no interests except Elinor, who quickly decided her aunt "seemed not to have developed beyond about fifteen." Elinor was soon as anxious to leave Hessle as she had been Kelowna, but Jeannie wasn't in any particular hurry to see her go. In a memoir called "London Life: 1930-1931," Elinor credited "getting on famously" with Jeannie's husband, Ivor, and conspiring with him to get Jeannie's Scottish terrier pup tipsy on port as the two factors that aided her second escape from family clutches.[4]

Jeannie accompanied her niece to London and stayed with her in the Regent Palace until Elinor could attach herself to a hospital. At the first opportunity, Elinor set off for the Royal Free Hospital in the hopes that Dame Louise would remember her from the Winnipeg meeting and suggest something. Dame Louise was operating but sent word Elinor could enter the theatre. Elinor did, and was astonished to see the great doctor wearing a pair of long earrings that dangled below her sterile cap. Dame Louise finished up, invited Elinor to tea, and referred her to the Annie McCall Maternity Hospital, saying she would call Dr. McCall on Elinor's behalf.

The Annie McCall Maternity Hospital has been described by doctors who knew it in 1930 as "primitive," "spartan" and "very individualistic." It consisted of two old houses joined together — that's where the staff lived — with an extension at the back serving as the hospital.

It was Annie McCall's personal fiefdom. Dr. McCall was thin, wore her hair pulled back in a bun and sported "clothes that never knew fashion."[5] The story goes that she kept the only pair of rubber gloves in the hospital locked up in her office. Although she left a large personal fortune when she died, this spirit of economy permeated the hospital. Staff made do with the bare mimimum in the case room, and were soon tired of rice puddings in the residence.

Dr. McCall, described as "a solid obstetrician in her day,"[6] trained nurse-midwives who were headed for Africa as missionaries. She believed that women in labour needed little if any anaesthesia; in fact the best thing for them was to be marched up and down stairs. She also, according to one former resident, allowed her time to be taken up with various "ploys" — such as a near obsession with ensuring total abstinence from alcohol among the staff. That sometimes meant that the day-to-day business of running the hospital came second.

Ploys and all, hundreds of Elinor's future patients would have reason to be grateful to the eccentric Annie McCall. It was in this "primitive" hospital that Elinor's hands learned much of their craft and skill. Over and over, Dr. McCall put her through the "phantom drill" — practising breech and forcep deliveries on a model of the lower female abdomen — until Elinor loved the challenge of safely delivering real breech babies. She learned Ritgen's manoevre — a technique of holding the baby's head while gently stretching the mother's perineum up and away from it to prevent the head from causing a tear. She learned a lot of things, she said later, "that were good common sense and . . . stood me in good stead throughout my practising and teaching career."[7]

Elinor was also sent out on home births, and this she enjoyed. The husband would come to the hospital with the news that his wife was in labour, and Elinor would set off for his house. The hospital was in a working-class district and the husband would follow about a yard behind her (presumably calling up directions), out of respect for their different social positions.

Elinor had personal as well as professional reasons to be grateful to the circumstances that led her to this small maternity hospital. On her first day she met a kindred spirit, to whom she later wrote of their friendship, "Someway or another you have found a key that only 2 or three people know exists."[8]

Dr. Isabel McGill, of Glasgow, was almost finished her six-month stint as house surgeon at the hospital when Elinor arrived. Heading up the stairs after breakfast, Dr. McGill found the landing blocked "by a figure standing still, bent double, apparently contemplating her feet."

"What on *earth* are you doing?" she demanded.

Elinor unfolded slowly and looked at the squarish figure confronting her. Why, it was Winnie the Pooh, or someone with an uncanny resemblance to him! She couldn't resist.

"I'm doing my stoutness exercises," she said, gravely.

Isabel was delighted. She later wrote, "Now a girl who would quote Pooh, on first acquaintance, and clearly expect to be understood, all in completely strange surroundings, was a girl after my own heart."[9] They had only a short time together, but the connection was solid and lasting. With infrequent visits to reinforce that connection, they had to rely on letters. They wrote, regularly and from the heart, for the next five decades. Like so many of Elinor's most cherished relationships, this one developed and grew on paper.

By the Christmas break, Isabel had gone back to Glasgow and Elinor was expected in Hessle for the holidays — a place where she could have used the support of her new friend.

Jeannie had been busy ordering herself and Elinor complete ski outfits, figure skates and "every other thing one could think of" for what, apparently, was going to be a "truly athletic holiday." Elinor later wrote, "Jean was not athletic, she had never been on skis nor skates, nor hikes but she was bound she was going to change all that now that she had a younger companion."[10] Jean chose Switzerland as the site for this transformation, and off they went.

The trip was a disaster. Elinor grasped the basics of skiing after one lesson but Jeannie was only humiliated by the attempt. Her bubble burst, Jeannie then, according to Elinor, "retired to the room with the sulks" for the rest of the holiday. Elinor, who had found a group of young people, managed to have a fairly good time and this only exacerbated Jeannie's bad humour.

Jeannie had cherished her self-image as a sort of Lady Bountiful/Pygmalion figure, and she had also invested heavily in the fantasy of madcap fun and recaptured youth resulting naturally from Elinor's arrival in her life. But Elinor had turned out to have no interest in being made over, or in frivolity, and what's more she had definite plans and ideas of her own. Elinor was cool to all suggestions from her elder and (therefore) better, and didn't even seem to like her.

Jeannie took this realization — and the loss of her illusions — badly. Just how badly was revealed at the end of a painfully silent train ride back to London. Jeannie abruptly announced that Elinor could stay in London as long as her money lasted but (in spite of her earlier promises) no more assistance would be forthcoming. Elinor was on her own. And she was not to visit Hessle again; she wasn't welcome.

It was a serious set-back, not the least part of which was

facing the reaction from her father, who had accurately predicted just such an outcome. Luckily, Elinor had gone to the Chelsea Hospital for Women while she was still at Annie McCall's to see if the Chelsea could take her on after Christmas. They had offered her a few hours a week in the Outpatient Department, but they didn't provide room and board. So Jeannie had found Elinor a room in a boarding house before the holiday took place. That was a bright spot, or at least one less thing to worry about. Best of all, given her new circumstances, was the discovery that the room had one really good feature: the lock on the receptacle for shillings for the gas fire was broken. Elinor could use the same shilling over and over to heat her little room.

Every cent she could save was a salve to her hurt pride. She wrote her parents that Jean was "making much cry of hard times and the money spent; . . . her tongue can certainly wound."[11] Fishing out the shilling yet again, she considered herself lucky to climb six floors to her room and share a bathroom (three flights back down) with 13 housemates. There were no kindred spirits to be found among them, unfortunately. Elinor described them as "very mouldy looking fixtures" given to frizzed hair and ostrich plumes.[12]

She must have written Jeannie a note saying she found her surroundings "nice." Jeannie sent back the crisp reply, "I quite expected Clauricarde House to be nice, I took a great deal of trouble over finding it for you." The next communiqué to the ungrateful niece read, "Surely you don't need to buy teas out — they are provided, and it wd be cheaper by tube to the boarding house — than buying teas out." The following week brought this: "Having every Saturday off must be rather nice it certainly shows you are not overworked; . . . of course you realize that it is due to *my* knowledge of hospitals and of my interest in hospital work etc. that the idea . . ." She thought Elinor *might* find the time to see the *wonderful* new radium clinic, one of the "sights of London!"[13] Elinor was both cast off and on a short leash. Perhaps her sense of obligation to her aunt, or a genuine desire to heal the break, kept her sending the notes and bits of news that only got flung back at her. An explosion seemed inevitable, but Elinor allowed the situation to simmer away. She had a great deal else on her mind because suddenly she was having an absolutely wonderful time.

Chelsea Hospital turned out to be perfect. Elinor sent a glowing report home at the end of January: "And so ends a busy & happy week; . . . it is glorious to get back to hospital again — I have been revelling in rubber gloves and the smell of ether once more! Chelsea is up-to-date in equipment — not archaic as Clapham was, & is a much larger hospital. I have seen some very good operations done by big men."[14]

Elinor's outpatient work took up only certain afternoons so she usually spent the mornings watching operations. One day, one of the "big men," Louis Carnac Rivet, took her along to another hospital where she could watch him do a "spectacular" Caesarian. Elinor later recalled that he did it in seven minutes, from knife-to-skin to the last suture. She was impressed, but she also tucked away the fact that such speed sometimes led to post-operative haemorrhage.[15]

She tagged along wherever she could, visiting hospitals and the clinics on Great Ormond Street, absorbing, watching, learning. But life was not all work. In fact, the first day she reported to Chelsea, a good-looking and "sprucely dressed" doctor showed up in the Outpatient Clinic apologizing for being "so far adrift," that is, late. As he was speaking, Elinor had a sudden (accurate) premonition that this man would ask her to marry him.[16] The name Bernard Collings began showing up so regularly in her letters home that her father finally remarked dryly that "this Dr. Collings" seemed to be "a particularly helpful chauffeur."[17]

Bernard was not without rivals. Elinor's father had given her a letter of introduction to a political friend of his, Sir Howard d'Egville. Described in the "London" memoir as shortish, balding and much concerned about dental hygiene, Sir Howard was not a romantic figure. But he was an exceedingly useful contact, and again Elinor's genius for attracting patrons as needed came into play.

Sir Howard was soon smitten with the "Prairie Flower." He took her to lunch at the Trocadero, dancing at Ciro's, golfing at Lord Roseberry's estate. They went to a levee at St. Stephen's Palace. Elinor's scrapbook contains her carefully preserved invitation to meet the Rhodes scholars at an "at home" hosted by Viscountess Astor. Another invitation came from the Speaker's House, Palace of Westminister. Elinor was living a fairy tale. She wrote in her "London" memoir, "I was indeed in the stratosphere!!" To which Aunt Jeannie could only sniff from Hessle, "What *do* you do! for dress. I can't imagine."[18]

This latest jibe from Jeannie was dated April 2. She had been engaging in intermittent sniper attacks since the Christmas holiday. At the same time, she disclaimed any responsibility for, or interest in, her niece's well-being. Elinor had finally had enough, and, judging from the letters that started flying in May, she must have blown up at Jeannie in no uncertain terms. And in writing. It appears that Jeannie, whose letters were not having the desired effect on her niece, was unable to bear the fact that Elinor was actually thriving without her. She raised the stakes. She seems, ludicrously, to have ordered Elinor out of England, threatening dire consequences if disobeyed.

Outraged, Frank entered the fray and sent two letters in as many days. In the first, he told Elinor not to be afraid of being forced to leave. "We think we shd not permit you to be despatched, unceremoniously, and under a cloud of recrimination from the shores of Britain." Warming to this theme, the second letter was stronger. He demanded, "Why should you submit to the treatment you are receiving and leave Britain like a chidden child. . . . I think it is a time to run the colors to the top of the mast."[19] He told Elinor to remember that she was the daughter of "two people who have not asked quarter or favors from any one and who, at least, are still able to pay the food bills. Now, go to it!"

In the course of the battle, Frank revealed quite a bit about his own childhood — one of "curses, epithets and blows" — under a tyrannical and abusive father. He felt that Elinor was being persecuted in a similar way by Jeannie, and wrote, "She is patterned after my father. . . . He never cd bear to see others happy and enjoying themselves. With diabolical ingenuity he used to think up jobs for me to prevent me getting off with other boys for an outing here or there. If my brothers and I were larking a bit in the kitchen (never where he was) "binf" wd go the bell."[20] In a vulnerable moment, with these memories revived, Frank asked his daughter to understand what he had had to struggle out from under. Then he pledged financial support, which couldn't have been easy, and "united love" from himself and Margaret.

If only he could have left it there. But his other side, his inability to let any mistake go unremarked — however sensitive the timing — made him turn around and treat Elinor like a chidden child himself. To put off delivering the following sermon would be neglecting his duty. His next letter listed the lessons Elinor could stand to learn from her experience with Jeannie. It reads, in part:

> (1) You entered into a loose arrangement and left the details to work themselves out later. When last in Kelowna you told us that Jean had remitted 60 pounds and that was all there was to it. You should as a matter of precaution have made your bargain in full at first. In consequence of the neglect to do this you suffered unneces-

sarily. Had it been otherwise you could have demanded the extra amounts which you did not get. The lesson of this is — *always make your business arrangements ahead of action.* Then stick to your side of the bargain at any cost, and *expect others to do the same....*

(2) You made a cardinal error in writing a letter while you were hot. *That is something you must never do, under any circumstances....* See what has happened in the present instance. You have armed Jean with a weapon which she can produce on any occasion that she wishes to ventilate her grievances. She has the documentary evidence to prove her case. And documentary evidence is irrefutable....

(3) The next point is psychological. You suppressed a complex. In that you, as a modern young lady, do not believe. You went on and on, took all the abuse or whatever it was from Jean, and just shut yourself up. The explosion was inevitable. People who are not contradicted come to believe that they cannot be, and become absolutely tyrannical in imposing their wills on others; ... it is a pity to have quarrelled with your benefactress and to have put yourself in wrong — in writing....

I would commend to you the psychology of the Master, which you will find in Matt. 18th. Chapter, and the 15th. 16th. and 17th. verses. Also In Matt. Chapt. 5, in verse 25. "Agree ... *whiles you are in the way with him.*" Which clearly means "make an early settlement before he has had time to go off and consult a lawyer." ...

Now a pertinent question. Are you altogether blameless in this matter? Was your attitude always such as would remove instead of intensifying a breach between you and your Aunt?[21]

The questions are fair enough, but coming as they did at the end of such a letter they virtually guaranteed that Elinor, proud and prickly as an offended teenager, would not take the hand her father clumsily tried to offer her.

She wrote Frank that it wasn't surprising Jeannie complained of her niece's lack of love and affection; after all, hadn't he and Margaret found her deficient in the same way? Hurt, she added, "Evidently I have just been myself over here." She went on to formally thank him for his offer. She said she was very well satisfied with her time in London and she declined to stay on at his expense. She told him that, of the 35 pounds she owed him, she had 12 on her. She ended the letter, "Sorry I am such a wash-out as a daughter! With love, Elinor."[22]

She was much more affected by what had happened than this flip closing remark indicates. In Elinor's collection of papers was a torn scrap that looks like a rough draft of an emotional letter to Ivor, Jeannie's husband. The writing is a scrawl — the ideas separated by agitated dashes.

> And so ends my year; . . . wonderful experience, do not know how to say thank you adequately. The hospital work came up — my expectations exactly; . . . social life surpassed even my wildest imagining. . . . E.B. should have mixed company — duchesses, aritsocracy [sic] . . . soon forget the thrill. . . . Oh! it *glorious* . . . am most grateful . . . my one regret . . . found me so lacking personally; no doubt due to inherent selfishness coupled . . . intensive scientific training. . . . On the eve of my return to Can. — leaving a bad taste in the mouths of all of you — I want to write special note "thanks"; . . . certainly I have not enjoyed playing . . . absolute ingrat-cad which has been thrust upon me merely because . . . one side unfortunate story has been heard. However, I trust the investment you have made . . . more truly thankful than I can express. . . . Swiss trip — it was 2 wks — absolute hell . . . hope . . . never experience anything like it again. No doubt if you ever did have a good opinion of me, you have lost . . . truly sorry . . . keep my mouth shut . . . best policy. . . . And so — many, many thanks.[23]

It's a little bizarre that Elinor considered laying partial responsibility for the quarrel with her aunt at the door of her "intensive scientific training." On the other hand, that training and what it had cost was very much on her mind. In the midst of this familial unheaval, Bernard had proposed — and in no less romantic a setting than Anne Hathaway's cottage.

Elinor wrote in the "London" memoir that she thought very seriously about accepting. But Bernard was from an aristocratic Guernsey family. He said his people wouldn't tolerate him having a working wife. And they weren't the only ones.

Elinor couldn't have been unaware of the Depression-inspired backlash that had already begun against married women who worked. *Maclean's* magazine ran an article describing such women as selfish, shameful and "a menace to society."[24] In Manitoba, the province that had been first to give Canadian women the vote, the government banned the employment of married women in the civil service. What about the 18 married women already employed by the provincial government? Each case would be investigated individually and "perhaps not all [the women] would lose their jobs."[25] The hunt was on, and it would get worse.

And yet Elinor had, at considerable expense, been in training for years. To work. She couldn't justify giving it up. She thought about a remark that Donald's wife had made to her as she was entering medical school. Lucy had said, as a compliment, "Elinor, I give you five years before you're married." Elinor had laughed it off then, retorting, "What would I do with a man in the kitchen?" Now, six years later, it wasn't so funny.

She wouldn't give up her work, but she couldn't break it off with Bernard either. They concocted idealistic and hopeful scenarios. One idea was that Elinor would build up a thriving practice quickly, say within a year, then sell it and return to England. After all, she was not just another newly graduated GP; she had "done" the London hospitals. The extra experience, while it conveyed no special title, was bound to help her attract patients. The best part of this plan, Bernard reasoned, was that Elinor would have had a taste of practice and wouldn't be given to recriminations and regrets later. Her training would be vindicated, her abilities proven — and they could marry. "Ah, youth!!" Elinor wrote, a bit ironically, in the Stoughton memoir.[26] These engrossing discussions served only to make her remaining days with Bernard slip away even faster.

The last day came. Elinor wanted to go and say goodbye to her benefactor, Sir Howard. Bernard wasn't enthusiastic but agreed to take her to Sir Howard's office. He told her that if she wasn't out in 15 minutes he was coming in after her. From the office window, Elinor could see him, bowler hat and furled umbrella, pacing up and down.

She said goodbye to Sir Howard and made it out in time. As for what passed between her and Bernard, she later wrote only that their final leave-taking was in a taxi outside the boarding house. A friend of Elinor's was waiting inside, prepared if necessary to cope with a flood of tears.

But only a trace of any of this appears in Elinor's last letters home. Once, she mentioned an outing with Bernard and followed the remark with, "I could weep when I think of leaving London!"[27] Apart from that, she showed her parents only confidence.

She wrote, "Winnipeg will be my sphere."[28] She rejected the idea of saving money by living with them in Kelowna. She said she was better off where she was known. She went on, "Also I have applied for a part-time demonstratorship in the Anatomy Department and as I do not see why sex would be a barrier there, I am reasonably sure of an appointment, with $500 attached. Then while I am looking about during the summer months I can do the Y.W. examining which nets me anywhere from $5 - $13 a day."[29]

The part about the demonstratorship in anatomy was sheer bravado. Elinor had known since February that the position was anything but definite. She had received a letter from Dr. MacLeod, secretary of the Medical College, informing her that little would be decided until a new chair of anatomy could be found. This was proving quite difficult, so much so that Dr. MacLeod even suggested in his letter that if

Elinor happened to run across a "first-class man" she might tell him to apply. But, he stipulated, "We are not taking an American."[30]

Elinor decided to spare her parents these details, and simply give them her final word on the subject of Winnipeg — "I want to get on my own at any price."[31] In the months that followed, as she sat in a silent basement office looking at an empty waiting room, in a city where staggering numbers of patients (and some colleagues) were on city relief, she had ample time to think about the price.

Four

STRUGGLE

▼

I honour the male, in all things but marriage. Yes, with all my heart I am my Father's child. (Athena in Aeschylus' Eumenides)

I was indeed my Father's daughter! (Elinor Black)

June 27, 1931

My dear Black,
     We had a call from your daughter, the "Doctor," and she told me that she intended to start practising in Winnipeg and the feeling existed that you would be coming to her rescue for funds to get her started. She showed quite an independent spirit in that she wanted to borrow the money rather than ask you to make the outlay. No doubt you will be highly pleased if her success is such that she can provide for a loan out of her fees. You will realize that a loan of this character is a difficult one for a Bank to grant and it would only be free from criticism if the collateral is beyond reproach. We know you can provide good bankable collateral, affording an adequate margin, and if it is your wish that we should assist be good enough to send us an endorsed note with securities duly hypothecated.
     Enclosed find the necessary forms.
     Eleanor said that she would require up to $1500.00.
Yours very truly,
J.S. Turner
Manager[1]

Elinor read the letter with mounting fury. When she'd sat in Mr. Turner's Bank of Commerce office a few days before, he'd shown nothing but kindly interest in her plans. And she, all business, had confidently gone out on the strength of the interview and seen about renting office space in the Medical Arts Building!

It was humiliating. If Mr. Turner had had doubts, why hadn't he expressed them to *her*, instead of writing to her father behind her back? Teeth clenched, Elinor turned to the letter her father had written to accompany Turner's.

Dear Elinor,
   I wrote you a "family" letter yesterday. The present is a business one and has to do with the letter from J.S. Turner, enclosed. There is no "banking" proposed in the proposition he makes, which is that, in effect, I advance my saving to you, while you pay the Bank interest for their use. . . .
   However, you have not taken me into your confidence as to your plans and you can hardly expect me to go it "blind" on the chance of losing something that both Mother and I may need very urgently one of these days.
   If the problem *has* to be solved by borrowing then I think it should come in small amounts. What would $1,500 be required for at one time anyhow? Would that be a maximum? If that amount be required now what assurance have we that you will not need more at an early date? If so, where is it to come from?
   Perhaps if you will discuss what you intend to do the way may become clear as to what suggestions I can make for you.
   Very cloudy and cool here, with occasional showers.[2]

Years later, Elinor realized that her father had suffered a greater humilation than she had. Frank was insulted that he, a prominent businessman and former minister of finance, should be asked to provide full security for a small loan. His signature alone, his word practically, should have been enough. It wasn't pleasant to learn otherwise, especially from a former colleague like Turner. Frank might be excused for feeling a bit fed up at repeatedly having his pride hurt and his advice ignored by his youngest daughter, and for sending such a cool message.

Later, Elinor would understand some of this. But the first time she read her father's letter all she felt was betrayal. In the Stoughton memoir she wrote, "I HAD told Father what I wanted to do and he had agreed to it. He should know that one can't start a business without capital and just on small amounts 'from time to time.' Now all my plans were in ruins."[3]

Totally distraught, Elinor headed like a homing pigeon for the Stoughton's apartment. If ever she'd needed a shot of unconditional love, it was now. It was a two-mile walk. She cried all the way there. It was bad enough being patronized by Turner but the thought of trying to set up a practice in Kelowna was worse — that rigid house, where she would always be "Babe," the rules, the fanatical housecleaning. By the time she got to the Stoughton's, she was crying so hard she couldn't speak. She just handed them the two letters and collapsed into an antique chair.

It didn't take Pater long to come to the rescue. He'd just been paid for his work on some University of Manitoba buildings. Within a few minutes of arriving, Elinor was looking through blurry eyes at a cheque for $1,000. End of crisis.

The Stoughtons wanted to make it a gift. Elinor insisted it be a loan, at six percent interest. That settled, the three of them indulged in the fun process (Elinor euphoric, Pater and Donna beaming) of deciding exactly how to best spend the money. Elinor would need a second-hand car, "but a good-looking one to create an appearance of success"[4] and second-hand office furniture and equipment.

Three days later, Elinor penned this reply to her father:

Your letter re my finances arrived on Friday, and was duly pe-
rused. I am so sorry that anything that would cause you and Mother
financial embarrassment has been even suggested. The obvious
thing to do is to drop the whole matter, to which end I have already
secured my capital from another source.

Things here are moving much faster than I had anticipated, and I
am greatly encouraged in my hopes for a successful career.

Elinor's signature from the time she was seven (and
forever after this one letter) had been and would be Elinor F.E.
Black. On this letter, however, she carefully dropped the *F* —
F for Frances — and signed off, "Your affectionate daughter,
Elinor E. Black, M.D."[5]

When she reprinted this letter in her Stoughton memoir,
Elinor followed it with, "I was indeed my Father's daughter!"
And she was. Of the six children, only Elinor, the last one,
was named after Frank. Frank had shaken off his own father
and risked a new country. Once in Canada, his spirit of
adventure had led him to bribe a train engineer to allow him
to ride outside the train, on the "cowcatcher" at the front.
Frank was petrified but exultant as the train screeched
through pitch-dark snowsheds in the Rocky Mountains.
Elinor probably felt the same way going it alone in practice,
at 26, in the Depression. The same drive that led a man who
left school at 16 to the provincial cabinet impelled his
daughter to break barrier after barrier for Canadian women in
medicine. In the Stoughton memoir, Elinor asked the reader,
"Didn't he know that pride of achievement and fear of defeat
was as strong in me as it was in him?" If he didn't, he soon
would, she implied, finishing her thought with, "I'd show
him!"[6]

At the moment, what Elinor and Frank had most in
common was pride — the stiff-necked kind. It was almost a
year before Frank could bring himself to ask his daughter
where she had got the money. By the time he asked, Elinor

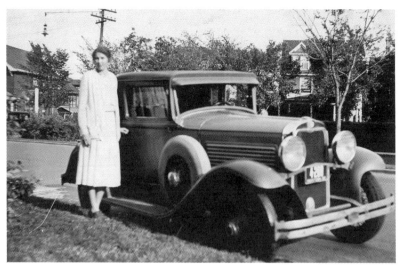

Elinor and "Teddy," her first car, 1931

had sold all the gold jewellery she owned to a dental lab for $32. When her sister Marjorie sent Elinor some dresses from the United States, it took Elinor 10 days to scrape together the $2.50 to get the clothes out of Customs. She lived on liver (at 18 cents a pound) and canned beans (at seven cents a tin).[7]

When doctors, including Elinor, reminisced about practising during the Depression, they invariably brought up the fact that city relief rates were one dollar for a house call and 50 cents for an office visit. What they didn't talk about too much is how they survived before the city relief scheme was in place. Elinor opened her office in July 1931. It was three years before the doctors won an exhausting fight to have medical care considered as essential as food and shelter and therefore covered by city relief. What did they do in the meantime?

Elinor, unaware of what she was in for, went out and spent half of Pater's loan on a Marmom "Roosevelt" roadster with red wheels and trim and a nifty rumble seat. She named it Teddy. She spent the rest of the money on furniture and supplies for her new office. Then she started to learn what her colleagues had known for a year.

The Outpatient Clinic (known as the Outdoor) at the Winnipeg General Hospital was for people who couldn't afford to pay for medical care. It was supported by general hospital funds; the doctors worked there for free. In 1928, 8,828 people had come to the Outdoor. By 1932, the number had risen to 24,582, and 80 percent of them were unemployed.[8]

One of Elinor's good friends from track-meet days was Bessie Pickersgill. Bessie worked as a dietician at the General, and she felt the small amount of relief money some people were getting was "just shocking." She remembered, "So we just met regularly and signed 30 to 40 special diets and then they got an extra ninety cents a week. . . . Once it was signed, it was a prescription for a special diet, they'd show that then when they went to get their Relief; . . . it was permanently upped."⁹ She signed hundreds of these "special-diet" cards for people who didn't need special food, just enough food.

Bessie also slipped Elinor sandwiches. Elinor was at the Outdoor four afternoons a week from 2:00 to 4:00. She wrote her parents that she was "tremendously bucked" to be asked. She looked forward to it eagerly each day and not just for the sandwiches. Elinor wrote in an article in 1936 that it was two hours she "would not have to sit in [her] office awaiting hopefully the footsteps that did not arrive."¹⁰

No one was going to see the doctor. People might *call*; in fact, dozens of people did call, all discouraging the doctor from coming to the house, all reduced to trying to cope with the help of some free medical advice over the phone. Even if a doctor did have patients, the situation wasn't much better. A Winnipeg Free Press editorial described the following as one doctor's "not in the least extraordinary" day at the office: "Twenty calls in one day. Of these two were of his own chronic poor cases, sixteen were on relief, one promised to pay and one paid."¹¹

The doctors started to organize. On December 10, 1931, there was a meeting of the Special Executive of the Winnipeg Medical Society. The meeting was held to take up the matter "of securing payment of medical men for services rendered to people on city relief."¹² The minutes show that the doctors felt that the load of providing free care for the numbers who needed it had become unbearable.

A payment scheme of some kind could hardly come too soon for Elinor. Her parents had gone to Italy where they hoped to ride out the winter more cheaply. At the age of 60, Frank had suddenly found himself unemployed, and, between real and paper losses, his estate was worth half what it had been in 1930. Pater was in trouble too. His business had slowed to the point where he and Donna decided to visit New York and investigate opportunities there. Elinor's receipts had been almost nil. For 25 cents a person, she was examining the feet (for athlete's foot) of applicants wanting to take swimming lessons at the "Y." She wasn't going to make it without another loan.

According to the Stoughton memoir, Elinor felt that this put her in a moral as well as financial dilemma. If she were going to marry Bernard soon, was it right to ask Pater for more money? Maybe Pater would feel that there was little point in such a loan. She wrote to him in New York and sounded him out on it.

Pater replied by saying first he hoped Frank's trip would not be too disturbed by the ignorance Elinor was leaving him in regarding how she was managing to live. Pater went on to confirm his love, his benevolence and his faith in his "dear childe":

> As to our own part in your business venture, we are glad to be able to lend a hand in such a good cause, as an expression of parental affection and the desire to have your effort succeed. You speak of the possibility of your bringing it to an end by getting married and we should be delighted to learn that this is to be. You will have carried on the business of your career far enough to show yourself and the world that your training and your own ability have been adequate. . . . Do not hesitate to let me know if I can make any further advancement.[13]

Dear, lovely, impractical Stoughtons. In fact, they were headed toward genteel poverty and soon wouldn't be able to make further loans. Perhaps they were wrong to mislead Elinor, but it *was* inadvertent — a negative response simply didn't exist in their vocabulary, even if it would have been kinder to give one. On the other hand, one can't put a price on the kind of moral support evident in Pater's letter.

What *is* a bit misleading, or at least one-sided, is the Stoughton memoir on the subject of marriage to Bernard. Elinor wrote the memoir in 1971, 40 years after she asked Pater about a second loan. While Pater's reply (November 1931) indicates that Elinor told *him* she was thinking about marriage, letters between Elinor and Bernard, and between Elinor and Sir Howard, give a different picture.

There were nine letters from Bernard in Elinor's papers. The first one is dated December 18, 1931. He pleaded guilty to being a poor correspondent but emphatically denied forgetting her existence. He also said, "I am truly and seriously alarmed to hear that Sir Howard is descending on you in your nice new flat in January. It sounds to me suspiciously as though your people might be 'arranging' things, in the pleasant way that Parents have." (Bernard obviously didn't know much about Elinor's history with her parents if he thought they'd be able to arrange anything that differed from Elinor's own plans.) Bernard suggested that Elinor tell Sir Howard "as a Great Secret" that she was already promised to another.[14]

However, a letter from Sir Howard, also dated December 1931, said, "I'm so pleased to hear you are not going to get married. Now that's a promise!"[15]

Bernard's first letter ended with, "Write soon and tell me how you are getting on. With best wishes. Yours, Bernard." That seems a little stiff for someone romantic enough to propose in Anne Hathaway's cottage. In his next letter, he reminded Elinor of that trip to Stratford-on-Avon. In his third letter, dated March 12, 1932, Bernard tentatively opened a discussion that one might think they should have had before Elinor left England. He asked a series of questions:

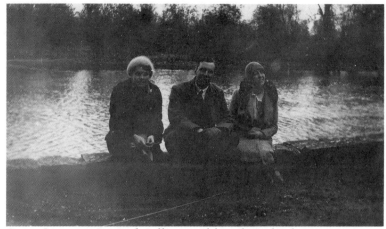

Grace Cameron, Bernard Collings and friend, England, 1931

Have you allied yourself with any male for £20 a month yet? I have been turning out my pockets to see if I can raise the necessary dollars to put in a claim, but am a bit fogged as to whether the £20 a month is meant to be just pin money only. . . .

How is your show progressing? It is a bit of a struggle, isn't it? Working up from nothing must be perfectly appalling. I wonder whether you have managed to raise the necessary ban this month, or if you are completely on the rocks by now. . . .

But seriously, do you ever think of getting married or are you too wrapt up in your professsion? Because, for a girl, getting married practically means dropping your profession, doesn't it?

Bernard went on to say that it was only fair he tell Elinor he "got pretty badly knocked about in the Service." He asked, "Would this make any difference to you supposing that our 'amorous advances' advanced any further?" After this oblique remark, he beat a hasty retreat, saying he didn't mean to be "previous" but thought Elinor would prefer also to be "out-spoken and candid." He signed off with a final query: "This letter would fairly make some of the old Folks' hair stand on end, wouldn't it!"[16]

Was the relationship between Elinor and Bernard really as delicate and tentative as this letter suggests? It's possible. Elinor's 1930 *Brown and Gold* university yearbook contains an article entitled "On the More or Less Gentle Art of Kissing." Directed at men, the article is full of admonishments — "The kisses a women gives you are beyond price"; and advice — "You don't have to teach a woman anything. Even if she has never ridden in a taxicab before, a girl has an instinct about those things."[17]

Elinor's memoirs indicate she went to London wrapped in this kind of innocence. In "London Life," for example, Elinor mentioned that Sir Howard kept telling her about his "trained cat" and that she should see it. She went to his suite for dinner, Sir Howard played "some very dreamy French" records and then invited Elinor to see the view of the city from his bedroom. Elinor found the view as ordinary as the cat had been, said her thank yous and left. She later wrote, "I walked to the underground station and took the train back to the South Notting Hill station wondering naïvely if Howard had had interior designs."[18]

Elinor drew an equally naïve portrait of herself when she described Pater's second attempt at nude photography. One Saturday, before the Stoughtons had left for New York, Elinor had gone to Pater's office carrying the kimono he liked her to pose in because the strong pattern showed up well. The office was all glass-partitioned rooms, with glass windows onto the hall. Pater suggested she take her clothes off, saying he'd always wanted to do nude studies of her.

Elinor was almost 27, a poised and self-assured doctor. In her letters to Charlotte, she was the ultimate young modern — hip, slangy and cynical. Some of the later Stoughton photographs are closer to "pin-up girl" than "sylvan childhood." But faced with this request from her benefactor, Elinor was like a child. She wrote in the memoir that she felt agitated, even "unhappy and frightened." She also said, "There was no pulchritude about me so why did Pater want to take pictures of my nude or draped body?" She worried about whether she was under "this much" obligation to Pater. All she could think of to say, finally, was that her mother wouldn't like it. She left, "as promptly as was polite."[19]

Elinor moved so confidently among men as a fellow professional; these anecdotes indicate she was at a loss if the relationship was anything else.

Naïveté is not the same as ignorance but it seems that, for a time, Elinor had to cope with both. Grace Cameron remembered her first visit back to Winnipeg after she was married. Elinor positively pounced on her for information, crying, "I've been waiting for you to come home. . . . These people

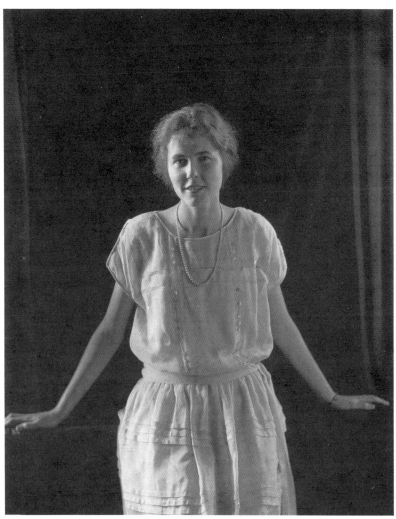

Photograph of Elinor by Stoughton, about 1926

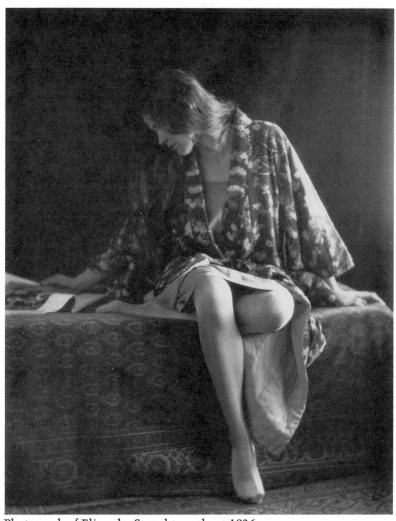

Photograph of Elinor by Stoughton, about 1926

[her patients] come to me for information. . . . I know nothing about intercourse!" Elinor added, "You don't get that in your doctor's books."[20]

Before she'd got married, Grace hadn't known anything either. It was her nurse colleagues who had told her how to make birth-control suppositories from boracic acid dissolved in coconut butter. (When the mixture solidified, it was like a wax that could be shaped and inserted.) Grace in turn shared what knowledge she had with her old friend.

It's amusing to picture Elinor sitting poker-faced behind her desk, desperately trying to think of some comeback to awkward questions from a new bride, all the while cursing the chauvinism that had kept female students out of MacKay's class on birth control.

It's a safe bet that her patients never suspected their doctor knew even less than they did. This was Elinor's worldly persona as presented to Charlotte:

May 3, 1932
My dear Larley —
. . . I bin shorta short a funds this month so I saved on postage stamps, that's why I ain't wrote.

Well, the family arrived this morning both looking very well — Mother has gained weight since I last saw her & looked very well. The old man is just the same. They both look quite prosperous 'specially the old man in a new suit. Fortunately I had cramps & diarrhoea — et sumpin as didn't agree with me — & when I got up this morning I sez to meself — "Splendid! you look all pale & washed out!" — & about the second word Ma said to me was "But Elinor, you are looking so white!" . . . I was afraid I wouldn't get any sympathy from the family. . . .

Boy! I've been splitting my sides laughing because Ma & Pa have raved so about Sir Howard's "courtesy," "graciousness," "thoughtfulness" & general attractiveness!!! The old bugger! I wonder what they would have thought of him if I had complied with his wishes to week-end with him! Isn't it a funny world? They say he is coming out in July & are quite bucked about him seeing me!! . . .

Also thanks for the bit on ski-ing — I can do it all, though. Clever, eh? You see in Suisse there are hills upon hills so you have to learn all those things before you move scarcely, or you will get going & won't stop until you either run into a barbed wire fence or the Mediterranean see?

I had my first baby 3 wks ago. It was Florence Howden's cousin, Mrs. McEachern's & boy! I hope I never have another like it. Not only was she not a good patient, but the baby refused to turn its head the right way. I stewed about her till I got fed-up & then got in a consultant. By the time the case was over, he said he had not had one like it for months & hoped he would not have another. . . .

In the middle of the tussle I thought "Well, if this is what I am up against for the next 50 yrs me for marriage!"[21]

But Elinor couldn't decide if she *was* for marriage. She had apparently responded to Bernard's hair-raising letter by suggesting they "re-open negotiations" in a year.[22] He didn't answer her for two months, which upset her, and when he did write, his reply was sombre. He explained that he hadn't written because he didn't know what to say. He added, "Women always claim it is their especial privilege to change their minds so the fact that you have always said you would never marry does not matter much. I doubt if I can stand my solitary state for still another year, but on the other hand I am rather afraid that until you have learned by bitter experience how 'un-rosy' earning one's living can be you would always be regretting having given up your profession and that would not lead to happiness."[23]

There it was again: the flat assumption that she would give it up. Every time she was faced with that attitude, she turned on her heel and went the other way. But she was confused; she gave out mixed messages. She sent Bernard a photograph of herself.

Society's message was clear. Winifred Holtby, in *Women and a Changing Civilization*, published in 1934, wrote this: "[Society] continues to track down those who do not marry

— (about 1 in 4 in modern England) and who do not have children, persuading them that their happiness is not happiness, their satisfaction not satisfaction, their preoccupations and interests a struggling and not too healthy sublimation."[24] Holtby wrote that women were relentlessly given the message that to live as an unmarried and therefore virgin woman was to live "under the shadow of a curse," with overwhelming pain and regret — the "psychologists, novelists, lecturers and journalists all [say] so."[25]

Bernard did not acknowledge the photograph. Elinor wrote Charlotte, "Sometimes I feel sort of weepy about it & other times I think that it wasn't meant to be & that is why I felt that I *could* live without him. However, as you know, it is sort of hard to get your mind all adjusted to the marriage angle, & then find that you have to change back & try to get the same old slant on your perfession, when you have discovered a whole lot of defects in it."[26]

She was also discovering some of the joy of it. In the same letter, she told Charlotte, "I had a baby on Thanksgiving day — a nice boy. Everything went swell & when I told the young pop about it, he was so jubilant I thought he was going to turn a handspring — he grinned all over his face & stuck his hand out & said 'Congratulations!' — so I sez 'same to you.'" Elinor told Charlotte that she had already collected $19.50 for the month and she was thrilled at the thought of covering her expenses by herself.

Bernard couldn't compete with such hard-won independence. He isn't mentioned again in Elinor's letters to Charlotte. His next message to Elinor was dated March 22, 1936. It consisted of three words on a single sheet of paper: "*Your turn. Bernard.*"[27] It wasn't meant to be.

Frank, on the other hand, was coming to terms with the fact that his daughter "The Doctor" was something that was meant to be. He would never stop trying to control her but for a short time there was peace. Elinor had won some respect from her father for doing it her way.

Elinor's parents had arrived back in Canada and came to Winnipeg for a visit; Elinor met them at the station. One of the first remarks Frank addressed to his daughter was a request for an appointment in her office the following morning. Elinor wrote in the Stoughton memoir that she sat regally in her swivel chair while her father looked around at what now amounted to at least $1,150 worth of debt. Elinor's gross income in 1931 had been $196.50, and 1932 wasn't going much better.

With difficulty, Frank asked Elinor if she would please tell him where she had obtained the money. Elinor told him, and Frank then asked if she was meeting her expenses from month to month. Elinor admitted that often she couldn't. Frank said he would like to contribute. Elinor didn't show the tremendous relief she felt, she just thanked him and "stipulated" that she wouldn't accept any contribution for any month that she did happen to make ends meet. When Frank left, presumably to do his duty by Pater and express a pained sort of thanks, Elinor, elated, wrote Charlotte:

> By gum! the old man has just been in & left me $85 worth of dividend cheques! Boy! it is a relief, 'cause the gov't has not yet paid Prf Stoughton, so he couldn't pay me & I was faced with having the 'phone cut off & losing Teddy if I did not get money by Saturday. You know there *is* a God! (Only two more payments & Teddy is mine!) The old man is in splendid form 'cause Man. is in such a mess financially that everyone here is saying to him — "If only you had remained with the Gov't - etc etc." — that sort of thing & you know how that goes over so big with him. Boy! — he'd give you the moon right now if you ast him for it. . . . A patient came in to pay a bill when he was in the ossif last night; I couldn't change a 10 spot so I ast him — he couldn't either but he had $5.00 which was the change I needed, so after the patient had went I sez "I'll go & get your

change now" — & he sez "You'd better keep the five dollars, you probably need it more nor I do!!!" I shure near collapsed! Fancy *him* saying a thing like that! So you see what a wonderful frame of mind he is in?[28]

After this encounter, Elinor loosened up enough to approach her father with a touch of her old mischief. She addressed a letter to him "F.M. Black, Esq. Financial Magnate" and signed it "E.F.E. Black, M.D. Financial Magnet."[29]

With her father on-side, Elinor set her sights on Donald. He and Lucy and their two children were also back in Canada. Donald had contracted tuberculosis in Korea and had gone to recuperate for several months in Kelowna. Now he and his family were spending a period of time in Winnipeg. Elinor was as obsessed with him as ever. She wrote Charlotte:

> I'm not making much headway with Donald — he's doing too much here — but I can't talk to him — I only get a yes or no or "I suppose so" out of him. I wonder, too, if he ever had anybody who knew the real him inside, 'stead of just the him he should be & seems to be. I have tried to pump the doctors who were in college with him & they all sort of say they didn't know him very well & he always had such high ideals that it kept him sort of above their level. One of them said Donald could be very unjust because his standards of living were so far removed from the average that he just couldn't understand ordinary human nature.[30]

Elinor was a student of human nature. She was drawn to psychology and theories about psychosomatic illness. She loved verbalizing her feelings and analysing motives. Donald's eluded her. She didn't understand religious faith. Frustrated, she complained to Charlotte, "He certainly can't be much of a realist if he goes preaching the Gospel in this day & age."[31] She attacked that part of his profession because he ignored hers altogether. He refused to discuss medicine with her. His monosyllables were a wall between them, and for all

Elinor prided herself on being a realist, she wasn't able to stop running into the wall and hurting herself.

A pattern, by definition, repeats, and family patterns are no exception. Elinor treated her mother much as Donald treated his youngest sister—as barely there, peripheral to the main story. In a rare mention, Elinor dismissed her mother as a compulsive housecleaner and "just so danged ornery and obstinate." Elinor asked rhetorically, "Boy! was I glad that the house here was sold — was I? — Now ask me. (Zat the right formula?)"[32]

Elinor lavished all her family love and affection and gratitude on Charlotte. She wrote Charlotte, "I shure do appreciate you — Bozo! Honest!"[33] She begged Charlotte to visit her in Winnipeg and dreamed of them renting a cottage for a holiday where she could spoil Charlotte and take care of her. Charlotte was the only one who knew how worried Elinor was almost all the time about money. Other close friends said later that they never saw Elinor discouraged; she showed them instead an "aura of nonchalant splendour."[34] They never realized she was in the same position as everybody else.

That is to say, terrible. In December 1932, Elinor budgeted 50 cents for "amusement." The Stoughtons could afford to give her only five dollars and two streetcar tickets for Christmas. When Elinor sat looking at her careful year-end bookkeeping she couldn't escape the fact that donations from Pater and her father outweighed receipts from patients and the "Y." Even *with* the paternal loans she hated, her total income still came in over $200 short of her expenses. She felt like "the champion family bum."[35] Would it ever get better?

Elinor couldn't look for help to the Medical Society's project for relief payments. The organizers were getting nowhere with the city, although, after almost a year, they had at least come to an official position:

> AND WHEREAS rent, fuel, clothing, etc are at present supplied at the public expense and not solely at the expense of those citizens supplying rent, fuel, clothing, etc.,
>
> AND WHEREAS medical attention it[sic] as much a necessity of life as rent, fuel, clothing, etc.,
>
> THEREFORE, BE IT RESOLVED THAT medical attention should be supplied on the same basis as other necessities of life, and therefore not solely at the expense of those citizens who supply medical attention.[36]

This position didn't cut much ice with Robert Jacobs, chairman of the Relief Commission. He sympathized but said neither the city nor the province had any money for the doctors. He wished them luck tackling far-off Ottawa. A delegation of doctors managed then to get an interview with T.G. Murphy, minister of the Interior. He promised faithfully to pass the issue to the minister of Pensions and Public Health or perhaps the minister of Labour or maybe the prime minister himself, why not? But the times were tough for everyone; the doctors shouldn't expect miracles.[37]

This was the general picture when "an old dame, aged 42 — unmarried, who had got herself pregnant" came into Elinor's office one day wondering if Elinor would give her "some pills." Elinor wrote Charlotte about the encounter:

> I ast her: "Why don't you get married" — "Oh! business is too bad & the baby would come too soon." "Well," sez I "get married anyway & go on working & don't say anything about it till later, then you have your certificate dated early enough so that the gossips have no come back." Sez she — "You mean a secret wedding?" Sez I: "I do" "Oh!" sez she: — "He wouldn't do a thing like that — he's much *too straight!*" Boy! I laughed — I just howled at her. Sometimes I wish I did abortions 'cause I turned down two this week — that's four hundred dollars gone to someone else.[38]

Four hundred dollars was twice what Elinor earned in 1931. Elinor took in only $550 from patients in all of 1932. Four hundred dollars was a lot of money.

Elinor was not tempted in the least. In a way, doctors who did abortions were protected by the community because they provided a necessary service. Everybody knew, nobody talked. But, in the event of scandal, the same community could be pitiless.

Shortly after Elinor had started medical school, a Manitoba judge had thundered, "It is the duty of the judge to pass a sentence which will act as a deterrent. Can it be said that seven years' penal servitude for a habitual abortion-monger is too severe? In our opinion it is not."[39] The judge wasn't even referring to the doctor in the case; the "abortion-monger" on trial was the woman who, for a fee, had told other women where to go for help.

Women who got abortions were considered by the courts to be victims, but that didn't stop judges from victimizing them all over again. One judge put it this way, "The victims of the illegal operations are accomplices in the crime."[40] Pity the "accomplice" in a different case — the doctor had performed the abortion, but first he raped her.[41]

In another case, seven pathologists were brought in to debate when the abortion had taken place relative to the woman dying of it. Five gave it as their "confident expert opinion" that it was two hours before death, the other two experts were convinced it was immediately before death.[42]

Reading the records of the abortion trials in the 1920s and 1930s is harrowing. The medical literature on the subject is worse. The women who could afford to go to the Medical Arts Building and offer Elinor $200 were in trouble, but they were also the lucky ones. The others showed up in the emergency wards.

The *Canadian Medical Association Journal (CMAJ)* published these case histories in May 1930:

A case I saw in the out-patients' department was an abortion self-induced with a piece of stove-pipe wire. The woman had aborted three weeks previously. Her legs were black to the knees with purpura. There had been two nosebleeds previously. Death occurred a few hours after admission. . . .

I was called to the medical wards to see a recent admission; the medical diagnosis was suspected ectopic gestation. I elicited the history of an induced abortion one month previously. The patient had been in service since, was not feeling well but was able to carry on. She then collapsed and was sent to hospital. When seen, she was bleeding from all the mucous membranes and purpuric patches developed later. Death followed in a few hours after admission.[43]

The next month the *CMAJ* carried a similar article. The author wrote, "Self-induced abortions appear to be increasing in frequency."[44] He described the things women took — quinine, castor oil, ergot, lead pills, pennyroyal — and the things they inserted, such as slippery elm, knitting needles and crochet hooks. Some women tried douches — lysol, potassium permanganate, vinegar, mustard, carbolic acid.

Into this bloody mess waded the birth control advocates. In Winnipeg, five local women's organizations, including both the Labour Women's Group and the University Faculty Wives, sent representatives to a meeting held to determine whether they should form a birth-control society. Providing birth-control supplies or information was a criminal offense carrying a penalty of two years in prison — unless it could be proven that one had acted in the public good. Many people involved in relief work were willing to take this line of argument, and the law was quietly but widely disregarded. One such worker wrote, "As president of the Women's Canadian Club, I was drawn into unemployment relief. My experience with those poor harassed mothers, with babies whom they did not want, could not clothe, made a deep impression on me."[45] She and others formed the committee that evolved into the Winnipeg Birth Control Society.

For a time it seemed that this committee, and others across Canada, risked having their agenda hijacked by the Eugenics Movement. Eugenicists were interested in birth control; in fact, they were terrified of being overrun by the hordes of children they believed born to "mental defectives" and other undesirables.

Dr. W.L. Hutton, medical officer of Health for Brantford, Ontario, president of the Eugenics Society of Canada, had this to say in 1933: "There can be no doubt . . . that the feeble-minded are increasing in Canada out of all proportion to the rest of the population." And the danger in that, another eugenicist pointed out, was that "those who make the country, who pay the taxes . . . are beginning to see that their taxes are being steadily increased by this immense burden of lawlessness, dependency, ill-health and incapacity."[46]

Some people who would never support legislation that increased women's rights could be swayed by an economic argument — often tinged with racism — about the wrong people having too many children, and the middle-class paying for it.

The lieutenant-governor of Ontario, the Honourable H.A. Bruce, used such an argument when speaking to the Canadian Club of Hamilton. He stated:

> At present Ontario spends annually $4,000,000.00 to maintain hospitals for the insane and the number of insane increases annually in Ontario so rapidly that every 20 months a new mental hospital has to be built for the accommodation of the increase. . . . At the present rate of increase in mental defectives, we shall within 25 years be spending $8,000,000.00 annually. . . .
>
> I have said on a previous occasion, and I shall always be of the opinion, that moral and religious sense necessarily revolt against the destruction of human life at any stage. But sterilization contem-

plates no destruction of life. On the contrary, sterilization means the ennoblement of life by damming up the foul streams of degeneracy and demoralization which are pouring pollution into the nation's life blood.[47]

That sort of frothing at the mouth must have made many thoughtful birth-control advocates decidedly uneasy. In Winnipeg, the committee supported a sterilization bill but took so much fire that members resolved to more or less drop that angle and get back to the main issue — how to get "scientific information on birth control to married women requiring it."[48]

The committee, which had officially become the Winnipeg Birth Control Society in January 1934, wanted to establish birth-control clinics run under medical supervision. The Winnipeg Medical Society was a little fussy about this, mentioning "certain religious orders" and deciding that they were "unable, as a Society, to do anything with the subject until such time as those who have initiated and sponsored the proposal have obtained legal sanction of their cause."[49] Thanks a lot, the women of the Birth Control Society might have said. They struggled on, and over the course of the Depression they helped thousands of families. But they never did manage to open a clinic.

Individual doctors could try to operate within the law, keeping ever-present the thought of the public good, and Elinor was one who did. She went further than the Birth Control Society; she spoke to unmarried girls. As always, she told Charlotte all about it:

Last night I gave a sex talk to the Norwood CGIT [Canadian Girls in Training]. Oh! I'm swell, I am — "such personality," "so frank" "so nicely put" — so I jest sez to all these sugary leaders — "When I was a CGIT girl I wanted to know a lot of things & nobody ever told me, so I made up my mind if I ever had a chance to talk to adolescents I'd tell them the truth without wrapping it up in a lot of sentimentality & bilge that only embarrasses them beyond reason." So I jest tells 'em fact & lets someone else to the moral & soulsaving part of it. Now I have done one church I shall probably be asked to do a lot more.[50]

Elinor loved teaching, and she was good at it. She also liked being invited to give talks because it was "the best kind of advertising," and if there were any paying patients left in the city she needed to find them. Her next letter to Charlotte revealed that she had had to stop hinting to the Stoughtons and ask for help "point-blank" and they had had to turn her down. She wrote, "Sometimes I just shudder when I think how my business would collapse if I couldn't get any more money from them & if pop couldn't afford to support both Mother's broken leg and me too. . . . I've only had one new patient so far this month — oh! I'm pretty blue for April."[51]

Forced idleness depressed her. She had to sit in the office in case someone did come. She wrote to Charlotte. She read — novels by H.G. Wells, and fiction and non-fiction by feminist writers Winifred Holtby and Vera Brittain. She thought up deals like offering to deliver her mechanic's wife's baby in return for brake repairs. She worried. She would have liked to smoke — but a woman doctor's office wasn't supposed to smell of smoke. She was always having to trip up the male colleagues who dropped in with lit cigarettes in hand. That was tricky; she didn't want to draw attention to herself as being any different from them, but she had to get them to put out their cigarettes.

With too much on her mind and not enough to do, Elinor got caught up in two crazes sweeping Winnipeg. One was benign. Overnight, apartments and homes sprouted card tables with half-finished jig-saw puzzles on them. Elinor would stay up until 3:00 a.m. if necessary to triumph over an "awfully muddled" puzzle. Such evenings only made it harder to stay awake at her boring office.

The other craze, while not exactly harmful, made a deep and negative impression on Elinor. A medical doctor named T.G. Hamilton was conducting sensational psychic experiments in Winnipeg. He organized hundreds of seances where different entities claiming to be R.L. Stevenson, David Livingstone, W.T. Stead or Camille Flammarion communicated through volunteer trance mediums. Photographs from some of the sessions reveal bizarre "teleplasms" or "ectoplasms" apparently emanating from the body of one of the mediums.[52]

Dr. Hamilton was a highly respected member of the community. He was a lecturer in clinical surgery at the University of Manitoba, a former member of the Legislative Assembly, former president of Manitoba Medical Association and a member of Executive Council of the Canadian Medical Association. There is no evidence that he was ever ostracized or ridiculed by his medical colleagues; generally, it was acknowledged that he applied scientific methods and rigorous controls to his experiments.[53] Mackenzie King, Sir Arthur Conan Doyle and others, well-known doctors, lawyers, musicians and writers, came to see him. In 1930 Hamilton lectured at Carnegie Hall.[54]

Elinor must have been aware of Dr. Hamilton. He was probably one of her instructors when she was a medical student, and from 1929 to 1935 he spoke regularly in Winnipeg about his findings. Not surprisingly, given his high profile, some people tried to imitate Hamilton's work or try psychic experiments of their own and Elinor become involved in something of this kind.

She never gave many details about what happened. In later years she mentioned she was "uncomfortably mixed up in spiritualism" for a while, but it scared her. She wrote, "Things I can't account for frighten me." She also said, "I will leave you with the fact that levitation DOES really happen."[55]

If Elinor had been looking to the other world for inspiration or advice on how to survive the Depression she didn't find it. However, tangible help from this world was on the way. On Febuary 13, 1933, Premier Bracken had stated, in writing, that "a *limited* expenditure for medical attention, *where* circumstances render such expenditure necessary, *might* be regarded as coming within the scope of the definition of direct relief.[56] Finally, on May 8, 1934, representatives from the City of Winnipeg and the Winnipeg Medical Society signed an agreement. The fee schedule was as low as it could be: 50 cents for an office visit; no operation could cost more than $25; a tonsillectomy was worth $10. So was a maternity case, and the $10 covered pre- and post-natal care and the delivery. No matter how many relief cases the doctors took on, the city would not reimburse over $100 a month.[57]

The doctors' reaction to this deal was euphoria. A 1974 article entitled "Sixty Years of Medicine in Manitoba" had this to say about the agreement:

> The doctors were almost delirious with joy. All felt that the occasion called for a celebration in the form of an evening dinner at the Fort Garry Hotel, to be complemented by an orchestra and a music hall type of entertainment — both to be produced exclusively by the doctors themselves under the general managership of the late Dr. Fred Young who was a patron and student of the living theatre. One recalls the orchestra of physicians, all rehearsed and conducted by Dr. Gordon S. Fahrni, with Dr. Tony Gowran as the First violinist. Numerous skits were presented on the theme of "Practising in Poverty," one of which in particular brought the house down. It was a solo act by a belly dancer who was billed as Mademoiselle Fluff-Fluff who rendered a routine of lascivious gyrations, being naked except for little more than strings of beads

strategically draped in a tactical arrangement. The supporting music was of the Tom-Tom variety and the dancer? — none other than Dr. Hartley Smith.

It was indeed a joyous party, but next day came the sobering if not shocking aftermath. Both newspapers roundly berated the shameful manner in which members of the medical profession had gloatfully celebrated the achievement of their financial coup in having cruelly gouged the poor taxpayers of Winnipeg.[58]

People on near-starvation relief, of course, weren't taxpayers and were likely to help celebrate this coup if it meant more secure access to medical care. Some of them, however, went a little overboard in their enthusiasm for the new arrangement. Either that, or they panicked in emergencies, but the result was often that, whereas before they couldn't afford to call a doctor, now they called three. It was *common*, one doctor groaned, remembering, to respond to a call in the dead of night, rush to the house — and meet a colleague just coming out of it. As the second doctor turned to leave, a third would be pulling up at the curb. Only the one who got there first was paid by the city. Competition was fierce.

Never mind. It was this agreement that enabled Elinor to survive, more or less. A hundred dollars a month was a huge help, but it didn't permit her to refuse her father's monthly contributions, gall that they were to her. Frank was once again playing the favourite family game — "Advice, Sermons and Home Truths."

First it was smoking. Frank asked her to resolutely set her face against "a terrible evil in womankind — as well as amongst male youngsters." Then he was off and running:

> I have no special interest in seeing you develop into a well-paid specialist, with a good income. That of course is in a measure desirable. But I do have a deep and abiding interest in knowing that you will fulfill your early promise of being a devoted Christian woman and a power for good in your community. The end of my years is approaching — perhaps more rapidly than I know — but it would be

a comfort to know that my daughters, who have all had much more advantages given to them than it was ever my fortune to have — are in the front-rank of those who are seeking to uplift their fellows. And, in spite of the Oxford Group and their cigarettes, I have yet to see the man or woman who has done very much for the Kingdom of God on earth with a cigarette between his or her lips. . . .

I do know I would be much happier to think of all my daughters able to say "No!" to cigarettes just as they say "No!" to liquor.[59]

Elinor scrawled "Oh! Yeah!!" in the margin next to this last line. She went on smoking and, presumably, drinking.

In another letter, Frank sent Elinor his analysis of her domestic arrangments. Elinor was sharing an apartment with Annie Taylor, a maternity nurse. There are some indications that Elinor was extremely attached to her. In the 1930 *Blue and White*, the student nurses' yearbook, the students published a "class will" where they listed lighthearted bequests to the doctors and interns they knew. To D.S. MacKay, Elinor's mentor, they willed a plaid apron to replace his pink rubber one. To Dr. McQueen, they left a fully armed guard for the nursery (perhaps to ward off paediatricians — there was a turf war over whose patients those babies were.) Elinor was willed Annie.[60]

Annie Taylor is mentioned again in a letter that Elinor wrote in 1959. This letter adds another element to Elinor's confusion about Bernard. She wrote a friend, "I left Bernard to come flying back to Taylor."[61]

It's impossible to know if Frank sensed his daughter's uncertainty about her sexual orientation, but he did send her this advice:

You have a problem on your hands with "Taylor" and are about to learn that friends — *as intimates* — *belong to periods* and are not fixed and constant. Your progress in your profession — indeed your living — depends upon wider contacts and, sad tho' it be, you may have to loosen some of the bonds that now hold you. . . . Do not permit any unsettled complexes to arise.[62]

It probably wasn't this letter alone that caused Elinor to lash out at her father. Circumstances had been more than trying for three years now. But this letter may have touched a nerve. Years later, Elinor had a terrible fight with Charlotte over the nature of Elinor's relationship with Gertrude Rutherford. At any rate, the truce between Elinor and her father was over. There's no record of the letter she wrote him, but it must have been scathing. Frank is bitter, almost vengeful, in his reply. His letter even came with a "warning ... not to be read at a time when you are tired or discouraged."

> Your letter, now before me, has a great deal to say about "independence," as being a family trait blameable upon your Father and Mother when displayed by any one of their children.
>
> As you have been, in a sense, "brutally frank," you need not object if you are repaid in kind. . . .
>
> The trouble with your reasoning is that you confound "*wilfulness*" with "*independence*." . . . If you wish an example with which you will agree, it was that of your Mother last summer when you thought her "difficult." That was simply because she would not surrender her will as to what *you should* do to *your* idea of what *you wanted* to do. . . .
>
> There is no such thing as "*independence*" in life. It is a compound of *pride* and *indifference*. . . .
>
> You have never in your life been able to be "*independent*," but you have been *wilful*. Without consulting me in the least you announced that you were about to start a practice in Wpg. You made no arrangements about future support. You placed yourself under obligations to others and when you were literally on the verge of starvation, due to your rashness, you had to turn to me at a time when the future was, for myself, most difficult and obscure. On that basis you have remained and it is only the extraordinary good fortune in obtaining results in a most speculative undertaking that has permitted me to go on giving you a measure of support. Under these circumstances "*independence*" is the last thing you have a right to speak of.

Ouch! Was it possible for Frank to say anything that would wound Elinor more? Yes.

> For how long is it *wise* to go on at a profession that steadily
> refuses to give you a living that prevents you extending actually, the
> slightest claim to *"independence!"* Had you become a stenographer,
> at a time when you worked for me in that position, you would have
> had a living wage out of it at least, or by now have been recognized
> as an *"able business woman."*[63]

Now that, as far as Elinor was concerned, was un-
forgiveable. It confirmed a fear that had always secretly
tormented her — people (men) didn't think she was smart
enough to be a doctor. Donald was the smart one, not "Babe."
Her brother wouldn't discuss medicine with her because she
was stupid. The money on her education was wasted. She
should never have aspired to anything higher than stenogra-
phy.

Elinor never forgot the remark. When she was at the
height of her success, she quoted it to journalists. She
included it in the Stoughton memoir, but not the loving,
anxious note Frank sent two days later. He never meant, he
wrote, that he would rather see her be a stenographer, just
that her profession was so hard, so draining. He asked her,
"Write all that is in your heart about it to me, soon, and we'll
decide *how* we are to see it through."[64]

Too late. All that was in her heart, once again, was the
determination to prove herself — and to the point where
what her father or anyone else thought wouldn't matter. She
was pushed a little further along this path by another of
Frank's suggestions:

> If you *must* continue to give free service to people why not give
> your life to it? I can imagine your life *invested better* in North Wpg.
> by living among people who need, but cannot pay for your help, than
> among those who can pay you but are indifferent. Personally I would
> rather contribute more — so long as I could — to work of that kind.[65]

So, her father would rather see her do missionary work, like Donald? Frank had "no interest in her developing into a highly paid specialist?" She would become a highly paid specialist. D.S., at the hospital, believed in her. He was urging her to go back to England and write the exams that would make her a Member of the Royal College of Obstetricians and Gynaecologists (RCOG). Those exams were gruelling. A stupid person couldn't pass them. Not many Canadians had their Memberships — and no Canadian women. If she went soon, she could be the first.

Five

GETTING THE "M"

▼

Good work. Shake. MacKay.

AMONG THE HARSH WORDS that had flown between Frank and his daughter was the interesting phrase "extraordinary good fortune in obtaining results in a most speculative enterprise." The enterprise was literally a gold mine. The mine, located about 25 miles south of Nelson, was called Kootenay Belle. Frank had held an interest in the mine for years; by 1936 the Kootenay Belle was producing, and the Blacks, as Elinor put it, found themselves "possessed of a welcome degree of moderate affluence."[1] In one later account, Elinor credited this turn of affairs with enabling her to return to England for more postgraduate work. Plus, she wrote, "I had taken my Father back into my good graces."[2]

Elinor wrote about the reconciliation in more detail in the Stoughton memoir. Her debt to the Stoughtons was weighing heavily on her conscience, she knew her elderly benefactors were hard up. She wanted her "M" (Membership in the Royal College of Obstetricians and Gynaecologists) very much.

And she believed she had to see Bernard in person to know, finally, what she felt about him. When Frank invited her to Vancouver, where he and Margaret were now living, she went, with all this on her mind.

At the same time, Frank had been thinking about his recent mild heart attack and the "iniquitous height of Succession Duties."[3] He'd decided to distribute Kootenay Belle shares among his children. He calmly conveyed this to Elinor as they strolled around the neighbourhood. Elinor almost burst into tears. The last six years had been so hard, financially and emotionally, on both of them. It looked like some peace was within reach. When Elinor found her voice, she told him about her plans, even about Bernard. She told him that her debt to the Stoughtons stood at $1,900 plus the $570 interest she insisted on paying. Within a few days, Frank transferred shares and arranged for her to send $1,000 to the Stoughtons. He doubted the Stoughtons' ability to handle money and suggested Elinor pay the rest in installments. In this he and his daughter were of one mind. Elinor, "wafted up onto a rosy cloud,"[4] started to think about England.

By June 1937 Elinor was almost ready to go. She spent $25, almost a month's rent, to have case histories of some of her patients bound into a book. She would need this later, to fulfill part of the requirements of the Membership. She also hired Dr. Marjorie Bennett, a recent graduate, to take over her practice while she was away.

Dr. Bennett was thrilled to be asked. She was in awe of Elinor at the time. She said, looking back, "[Elinor] was such a great person.... I just thought she was fantastic. I could have sat and listened to her for hours. Oh! I couldn't describe how I felt when she asked me."[5] Elinor flippantly told Marjorie she was hired because she didn't have frizzy hair. But the fact that Marjorie's two male cousins, also in medicine, had tried hard to discourage Marjorie from applying to medical school, may have had something to do with Elinor's decision.

The two women worked out an arrangement whereby Marjorie not only took over Elinor's practice but also moved into Elinor's bachelor apartment, had use of Elinor's car and stepped into Elinor's volunteer activities at St. John's Ambulance. Dr. Bennett didn't inherit Elinor's household help; Elinor didn't have any. Although she could now afford it, and hated housework and couldn't cook, Elinor told Marjorie that she didn't want an older woman around who might try to boss her.

Next, Elinor obtained a letter of introduction to none other than her childhood idol — artist Annie French Rhead. Elinor had made a new friend, Isabel McDiarmid, and on the walls of Isabel's home was, to Elinor's delight, Rhead's artwork. It turned out that Isabel's uncle knew Rhead personally. Isabel had also met her. Elinor hoped to exploit this connection and meet Rhead herself. Isabel had said Rhead was a fascinating gnome who truly believed in fairies. Elinor could hardly wait.

With all these loose ends nicely tied up, Elinor could concentrate on the most joyous part of the trip — her beloved Charlotte was going with her, and they were going to tour Europe for six weeks before settling down to their respective studies in London. Life was definitely looking up.

For this trip, and most subsequent ones, Elinor made her arrangements with Thos. Cook and Sons Agents. Cook's — "Our Couriers are socially acceptable"[6] — took good care of clients. The couriers attended custom and passport examinations with travellers, made reservations for them, transferred them and their luggage between stations, steamer and hotel, and handled the tipping. These elite employees were described in the brochure as "always in plain clothes, being quite a distinct staff from our [Cook's] interpreters in attendance at railway stations, ports, etc."[7] Not much could go wrong with Cook's in charge.

It was partly this firmly held belief that led to an incident on the part of the tour Elinor called "A Journey from Heidelburg to Prague in 1937."[8] The two sisters had been having a great time as Elinor, shades of *Perpetual Exercise Book*, recorded details like "S curve [on river] difficult navigation" and "hotel good but charged for jam." In most of Germany though, they were uncomfortable. They were often stopped and asked where they were going. Elinor wrote that they felt "very much aware" of Hitler's presence. Elinor and Charlotte were glad when it came time to leave Heidelburg for Prague.

Because their hotel was directly across from the train station there was no need for the usual Cook's courier. The women were on their own when the ticket-taker tried to convince them that their tickets were wrong. He wanted to re-route them. But he had to deal with Elinor's belief in Cook's infallibilty and her own intense dislike of unexpected changes in plans. The two sisters, each six feet tall in shoes, possessed of steel wills and intimidating manner, were insisting that they did have the right train and they were getting on it. The ticket-taker finally gave in and Elinor and Charlotte were led to a compartment.

They were immediately joined there by a man, carrying nothing with him, who sat and looked at them silently. As soon as the train got under way, a porter came in and pulled down the blinds on the windows. Elinor and Charlotte were annoyed all over again; they wanted to see the countryside they were travelling through. But this time they didn't argue. When they got to the Czech border, the porter came in and pulled up the blinds, and the man who had been sitting with them left.

Just before she and Charlotte left Europe, Elinor came across a magazine article about the German armament program. The article said that Furth-im-Wald, on the route Elinor had insisted on taking, was the centre of the arms industry and tourists were no longer allowed to travel through there.

The two women landed in England not as tourists but as students, and both good memories and uneasy feelings faded as Charlotte, at King's College of Social Science, and Elinor, in courses for RCOG Membership candidates, got down to work. And Bernard? Elinor said simply in the Stoughton memoir that she did see him again but he failed to sweep her off her "medically embedded feet."[9]

By November, medically embedded Elinor needed a break from the books. A day trip to see Annie French Rhead would be as complete a change of atmosphere as one could wish for, and with that in mind Elinor sat down and wrote to her. She promptly received an invitation to lunch.

The tiny, elderly artist and the tall, young doctor met at the train station in Kenley. Elinor was enchanted with her hostess, whom she described as puckish and utterly haphazardly dressed. They walked some distance to Rhead's home, which sat surrounded by a huge garden. Rhead lamented that it was November and all the fairy places were looking so drab. Elinor had the feeling the garden was loved, but not "cared for" in the normal sense. She promised to return in spring.

The visit was a great success except for one thing. Elinor could not stand being cold. Her friends suffocated at her place in Winnipeg — one was driven to playing bridge in her slip. They suffocated in their own homes too, if Elinor came over. Unless they turned the heat up, Elinor wouldn't take her coat off. In the four-page account she wrote about her first visit to Rhead, Elinor mentioned being cold, or frozen, or congealed, no less than 14 times. Although she was trying to concentrate on how delightful and intriguing Annie French Rhead had turned out to be, she was distracted by the fireplace. Elinor surreptiously studied it, deciding with despair that it was "thermally all wrong: the fire box was placed too far back."[10] Somehow, Elinor survived until train time.

A few weeks after this visit, Elinor learned she'd obtained a six-month appointment as house surgeon at the South London Hospital for Women. This stint was also part of fulfilling her Membership requirements. She'd get a small salary, plus board, residence and "ordinary laundry." Charlotte left England at Christmas to start a master's degree at Columbia in New York, and Elinor moved into residence. On January 1, she took up her new duties.

The South London was as different as a hospital could be from Winnipeg General. One letter among Elinor's papers indicates that women were not allowed on staff at the General in the 1930s. (A contemporary of Elinor's demurred, saying "I don't know whether it [was] a matter of being allowed. I don't think there were any. I think it was a matter of custom."[11]) The South London, however, which had several departments besides obstetrics and gynaecology, was built with the advancement of women doctors in mind. In 1912, a group of anonymous donors provided £53,000 to build the hospital, and another £40,000 as an endowment provided that the hospital "could be certain always to be officered by women doctors, and to admit only women patients (no males over the age of six)." The final stipulation was that the donors would remain anonymous forever.[12]

By the time Elinor arrived at the hospital, anonymous donors had paid for 40-bed extensions, a new outpatient department, equipment and a new nurses' residence. Dr. Margaret Louden, Elinor's supervisor at the hospital, recalled that "women patients anxious to be treated by women doctors came from all over the country, and such was the enthusiastic support, it [the South London] was one of the very few voluntary hospitals that was always solvent."[13]

Dr. Louden described Elinor as assured, in full command of her subject, shrewd and humorous. Elinor wrote that the hospital was a happy place. Because of her six years in general practice, the younger women considered her a fount of all medical knowledge. Elinor in turn relied on them to interpret the British system. She never really got used to her chiefs being rather distant. They didn't welcome calls from house surgeons unless it was a dire emergency, whereas Elinor had been accustomed to easy and continual consultation with MacKay, McQueen and her other mentors back home. At South London, one of her chiefs told Elinor she would have to do a thousand pelvic exams before she could be expected to find any mass smaller than a turnip.

It's doubtful Elinor had quite that much experience when she faced her Membership examiners in April. But she was ready. She wrote the two three-hour exams consisting of three questions each. Each question was worth 25 marks. Under observation, she examined a patient in the hospital. That was worth 75 marks. So was the 45-minute *viva voce* exam. Out of the 300 marks total, she had to get at least 225, but if she failed in two parts, she would fail the whole exam, even if her overall mark was better than 225.[14]

But of course she didn't fail. She sent the good news to D.S. MacKay, the man who had pushed her to try. She treasured his three-word cabled reply: "Good work. Shake."

Part of that good work had been done before Elinor left Winnipeg and had been presented to the examiners in the form of the expensively bound case histories. Elinor detailed 25 obstetrical cases and 10 gynaecological cases. They are a fascinating record of both birth procedures and social attitudes. In one case, a badly deformed expelled foetus was matter-of-factly referred to throughout the history as "the monster." In other cases, Elinor evidently found it noteworthy that one patient was "obviously of breed blood" and another didn't live with her husband and "her mode of making a living was questionable."[15]

There are several mentions of "criminally induced" abortions in the case histories. In one, a 20-year-old had inserted slippery elm. After the patient had been in hospital for 15 days, Elinor decribed her as looking "extremely toxic." The woman recovered a few days later, but Elinor kept her in the hospital an extra three weeks. Elinor explained in the case history that she did this because her young patient was a waitress who would have had to go straight back to work "if she was to have food and shelter."[16]

Elinor's obstetrical patients were guaranteed hospital food and shelter for at least 10 or 12 days after giving birth. After all, a maternity case history read like this: Pelvic Measurements, Obstetrical History, Menstrual History, Previous Illnesses, Present Illness, Labour. The present illness was the current pregnancy.

One of Elinor's patients obviously thought that this was nonsense. Under Present Illness, Elinor had been forced to write, "Patient was first seen one week before delivery; she had been feeling well all through her pregnancy, and saw no reason why she should see a doctor until the baby was due." The birth was "entirely uneventful" and under "Follow-up Exam" Elinor could only state, "Patient resumed her disbelief in doctors and did not report."[17]

Once in medical hands, however, the healthy sceptic would have gone through the same routine as other women. This is what Elinor wrote about a typical birth at Winnipeg General:

> When in labour the patient is admitted to the Waiting Room of the Maternity Ward; she is put to bed and given a full sponge, after which the pubic hair is completely shaved. In some cases the abdo-

men, thighs and perineum are painted with mercurochrome and acetone solution, but this is not done routinely. Following this, the patient is given two soap suds enemata, about one hour elapsing between the treatments providing the labour is not progressing too quickly. . . .

When the woman is ready for delivery, she is moved by stretcher on to the obstetrical table in the Case Room, and an interne is in attendance to administer a few drops of chloroform and ether (1:2) anaesthetic with each pain, and to encourage the patient to make good use of the uterine contractions. She is then draped with a sterile gown, stockings, and sheet, and the vulva is thoroughly washed with a 5% lysol solution. . . .

Following delivery and washing-up, tight abdominal and breast binders are applied, and the patient is removed to a warmed bed in the Ward. A drachm of an ergot preparation is given by mouth, and an ice-cap is applied to the lower abdomen. The ergot preparation is repeated in half-drachm doses thrice daily until six doses have been given. . . .

From the third post-partum day, the patient is turned in the prone position for one-half hour twice daily. . . . Providing the mother's condition warrants it, and her puerperium has been uneventful, she is allowed to have a backrest in bed on the eighth day; out of bed on the ninth or tenth day, and is discharged on the eleventh day or twelfth day.[18]

Former labour-floor nurses recalled that some of these new mothers, upon being discharged from the hospital, had to be wheeled out to waiting cars or taxis. After 10 days motionless in bed, the patient's legs were like jelly.

On a maternity ward in the 1930s, before infection-fighting drugs were widely available, a little lack of muscle tone in the legs was not considered a serious problem. Sepsis — "childbed fever" — was. Women died. Sometimes healthy women, with normal pregnancies, who came in for "entirely uneventful" deliveries, died. In 1928, a Winnipeg editorial used the phrase "this slaughter of young mothers."[19] Ten years later, the Manitoba Medical Association Review warned that whatever was going wrong was going more wrong every year, that all interference with normal labour was risky, especially in "the hands of the average" and teachers must make sure not to convey the impression that "certain operations or analgesias are perfectly safe, to be undertaken whenever the doctor finds it convenient."[20]

Between 1931 and 1940, 124 Winnipeg women died puerperal (the period just after childbirth) deaths.[21] Elinor saw this happen often enough. When she was preparing her case histories for her "M," it happened to one of her patients.

Mrs. C. was 27 years old, expecting her second child. The birth of her first baby had been free of problems, and under Present Illness Elinor had written, "Patient was very well throughout pregnancy." Mrs. C. went into labour at seven in the morning; by mid-afternoon, she gave birth to a daughter, seven pounds, four ounces, condition good. Half an hour later, Elinor noted, "Spontaneous expulsion of placenta and membranes intact. No laceration. Bleeding normal. Condition good."

Two days later, "No complaints." But the next day, Mrs. C.'s temperature started to rise. Three days after that, she was transferred off Maternity so the infection wouldn't spread. Four days later, the first dose of animal serum was given. This serum had been developed by a bacteriologist, using rabbits that had been inoculated with bacterial organisms likely to be implicated in the infection. The next day, Mrs. C.'s temperature was way down and she was feeling better. But the following day it shot up again. More animal serum. Three days later, her temperature was 106. In spite of that, the mother showed a keen interest in her baby, who was gaining well. But the next day, Mrs. C. started slipping in and out of rationality. Sometimes she could talk, or read the paper, sometimes she had to be put in restraints. Animal serum was given every day but on the twenty-third day Mrs. C.'s pulse was 160. Elinor wrote, "Her condition is completely hopeless." On the twenty-fifth day — "Patient cannot speak."

And on the twenty-sixth day after entering the hospital as a strong and healthy young woman, Mrs. C. "ceased to breathe" at 2:15 in the afternoon.[22]

Mrs. C. was a victim of one of the worst outbreaks of sepsis the Winnipeg General ever experienced. She was one of four women who succumbed simultaneously to a streptococcal puerperal infection. The maternity ward was closed to new admissions and the four women were isolated. But a few days later, four more women showed signs of infection. Five of the eight women pulled through. Of the three who died, two were in a weakened condition before they entered the hospital. But Mrs. C., Elinor wrote, represented "the ultimate tragedy of puerperal sepsis occurring in a healthy patient following a normal and uncomplicated delivery."[23]

The maternity wards were closed for two weeks and scrubbed down. Those who were around at the time as students or hospital personnel recalled that the epidemic was kept very quiet. All nurses, doctors and interns took to wearing masks whenever working with a patient in any way. All the sterilizing equipment in question was thoroughly checked for defects; none was found. The source of the infections, Elinor wrote, was never identified, but she believed it was undoubtedly "the nasopharynx of some person or persons attendant on the patients."[24]

Six months later, prontosil, the first of the sulphanomides, became available in Winnipeg, and Elinor used it to help save the life of the young waitress suffering from a septic abortion, self-induced with slippery elm.

The experiences detailed in the case histories marked and shaped Elinor's attitudes for years. Fear of infection influenced her feelings about Caesarian sections. Fear of infection was one of the main arguments for building a new, completely separate maternity pavilion in Winnipeg; Elinor, in addition, always tried to keep gynaecology patients out of it.

Given her experiences, one wonders what Elinor's reaction was to having to undergo surgery herself, just before she left England, and to the strange note she received while in hospital. Elinor had her appendix removed, and an acquaintance was prompted to write, "I have the Hospital list, and see that you are to have the operation this afternoon, so that it will be all over by the time you get this, and I do so hope you will not have too bad a time and that you will even be able to look back on the time as a happy experience, as I certainly can do myself about the various operations I have had."[25]

That seems a dubious hope, and at any rate it wasn't Elinor's custom, yet, to spend time looking back at anything. She had prepared her case histories, done the work, written the exams and was returning to Winnipeg a specialist, the proud and only female Canadian owner of five letters: MRCOG — Member of the Royal College of Obstetricians and Gynaecologists. She was looking forward.

That was definitely the impression Elinor gave when she addressed the University Women's Club luncheon upon her return to Winnipeg. Perhaps the spirit of the South London was still fresh in her mind — she gave a historical rundown of women in medicine. She mentioned Dr. James [Miranda] Barry, a woman who dressed as a man to get into medical school. The disguise was successful — Dr. Barry spent her entire medical career in the military; in 1857 she was appointed inspector-general of Hospitals for Upper and Lower Canada.[26]

Elinor also named Elizabeth Blackwell, Emily Stowe and others. She talked about the women doctors who were first, about the ones who started hospitals, about medical women in Spain and France and Germany and the United States and Canada. What she was trying to do, according to her lecture notes, was prove that women doctors were neither "species of *rara avis*" or "biological aberrations."

Elinor convinced at least one woman in the audience. This listener recalled, decades later, "We were kind of spellbound. I remember that lunch vividly. I was fascinated with this young person." Elinor, "full of vim and vigour," left her audience with the distinct impression that she just "wanted to get going now — to make her mark."[27]

▼ Six ▼

HEARTBREAK
AND LOSS

▼

Blessed is she who has found her work; let her ask no other
blessedness. She has a work, a life purpose; she has found
it and will follow it! (Thomas Carlyle, pronoun changed)

SMALL WONDER that Elinor compiled a list of names of
women doctors and their accomplishments and then spoke
the names out loud at the women's club luncheon. If Elinor
had been introduced to the concept of mantras or affirm-
ations, she may have felt like intoning *Barry Blackwell*
Stowe as she went from office to hospital. Because as it was,
in her present surroundings, it was almost impossible to find
herself reflected. A newspaper item calling attention to her
status as the first Winnipegger to obtain the "M" also mentioned that Elinor was "the only woman lecturer in a medical
subject in a general teaching hospital in Canada."[1] The only
one. What must that have been like, especially after the all-
women medical teams she had just left in England?

Elinor's feelings about her situation at the Winnipeg
General would have been complicated further by the way

women were presented in popular magazines such as the *Canadian Home Journal (CHJ)*. Just as Elinor was returning to Canada, *CHJ* did a survey of the 1938 "girl" graduates from McGill, Queen's and the University of Toronto.[2] Posing the questions, "Has it [university] made her intelligent or merely critical?" and "Is it worthwhile to send a girl to college?," the survey questioned 169 new graduates. *CHJ* found that the majority aspired to secretarial work, with teaching coming second and journalism third. (Alice Harriet Parsons, who wrote the article, reacted to this last by saying, "I'm afraid there are going to be some disappointments here — there just aren't fourteen openings for girl journalists this year, or any year.") Medicine wasn't mentioned at all as a career.

Marriage and children did receive prominent mention — 166 of the 169 respondents defended themselves against "accusations of race suicide . . . hurled at college women" by declaring that they wanted more than one child. And 91 percent said they asked "nothing better than the chance to give up their job and settle down in a home of their own. With the right man, of course."

The ads surrounding articles like this one illustrate the advertising industry's opinion of women. One ad was directed at prospective fathers: "Just as soon as his wife believes she is going to have a baby, the modern husband should get in touch with a competent doctor who can give her first-class care. Then he accompanies his wife on her first visit to the doctor's office, giving her added confidence, answering many of the doctor's questions and receiving the medical information."[3]

First, though, it was necessary to get that husband, and one hysterical ad gave the following warning, "Unpopularity often begins with the first hint of underarm odor. This is one fault that men can't stand — one fault they *can't* forgive. . . . Smart girls — popular girls — don't take chances! They know a bath only takes care of *past perspiration* — that they still need Mum, to prevent odor *to come.*" Those women who had husbands and children could contemplate another ad, one featuring Shirley Temple: "Doesn't Shirley's breakfast of Quaker Puffed Wheat look simply delicious?"[4]

Women having babies kept Elinor in business, and she was hardly against it, but where did she fit? Obviously not in any world portrayed by *CHJ*, and a professional journal, *The Canadian Doctor*, didn't welcome her with open arms either. While Elinor had been preparing her case histories for her "M," *The Canadian Doctor* had run an article called "Women in Medicine." The article worried that the number of women doctors had passed the "saturation point" but then reassured readers that women would never "contend with men in the medical profession . . . largely for the reason that they are women. Physically alone they have not the strength or the constitution to stand up against the continual strain and the hard work."

Moreover, the article went on, "women rarely exhibit that independence of action or breadth of viewpoint necessary for the carrying through of big and important work. They lack a sense of relative values which results in obscuration of the main end by a number of minor issues." Being faced with a different point of view had really irritated the author, or authors. (The article was bravely signed "Say Men.") Like Henry Higgins, "Say Men" deplored the inclination of women to be women and not men. Women, apparently, tended to "seize a point of small interest and develop it out of all proportion to its value."[5] The article didn't give any examples of differences in male and female values.

Another article did tackle that question, as well as some of the other points raised by "Say Men". This article, by Stephen Spencer, ran in the *Saturday Evening Post* under the title, "Do Women Make Good Doctors?"[6] Despite the silly question, and the occasionally patronizing tone ("forthright little lady doc"; "a gal with gumption enough to gather up her new-look skirts and jump"), Spencer's article exposed several examples of, to him, "amusingly transparent" sexism.

He made fun of the New York Obstetrical Society's "logic" in not admitting women as members because it held meetings at the Yale Club and women weren't allowed in there. He challenged the argument that taxpayers' money was wasted on producing women doctors who would only get married. Spencer quoted the results of a poll that two women professors had undertaken of 1,240 women who had graduated in medicine between 1920 and 1940. Over 90 percent of the graduates were in full-time practice or teaching or research. Of the 451 women doctors who married, 82 percent were practising medicine.

Spencer also quoted Dr. Ann Preston, Quaker dean of the New England Female Medical College in 1848: "We must protest, in the sacred name of our common humanity, against the injustice which places difficulties in our way, not because we are ignorant or pretentious or incompetent or unmindful of the code of medical or Christian ethics, but because we are women."

Spencer wondered why, if the medical school deans were right about there being no quotas, the proportion of women students never got above four or five percent. And he pointed out that there were 1,102 hospitals providing residency training, but only 318 took women graduates.

As for the women doctors' lack of "a sense of relative values" that so discombobulated "Say Men," Spencer quoted a doctor in Elinor's own field. Gynaecologist Catharine Macfarlane spoke about preventive medicine, comparing it to good housekeeping. "You have to keep at it," she said. "You can't let it go and then do it all at once." Macfarlane added, "I think women physicians are quick to appreciate this point of view, and to insist that things be taken care of while they are minor, rather than allowing them to become advanced and serious. Preventive medicine requires a lot of painstaking and unspectacular work, which women are good at, but it will be the medicine of the future."

Elinor could have used the support of Spencer's article 10 years before it appeared. By the time it did, in 1948, Elinor was successful, a rising star. But in 1938, she was struggling, caught between the ideas in *CHJ* and those in *The Canadian Doctor*. Around 1938, "Say Men" were insisting that, even though women had been "freely admitted" to medical schools for "so long, . . . not one [had] been outstanding." Not one had ever "at any time seriously challenged male supremacy in the world of achievement."[7] *Miranda Barry, Elizabeth Blackwell, Emily Stowe* . . . and Elinor? A friend recalled being in Elinor's apartment "with coffee perkin' on the gas" and Elinor saying "Kinney, you know, some day . . . "[8]

Elinor had her list — and her hopes — and she was holding fast to them. A second attempt at a relationship with a man was not working out. Lieutenant-Colonel Orville Kay had honourably stood aside while Elinor saw Bernard a final time, but now Kay was declaring himself. He sent Elinor "hearty congratulations" on her success in England and told her D.S. MacKay was more excited about it than his telegram had conveyed. Kay wrote that MacKay told him, "You know people have been saying I worked the girl too hard — but damn it I had to show the old fossils around the hospital that she could do a man's work better than a lot of them could." Kay also wrote that D.S. and other people thought Elinor was just about perfect.

By the end of the letter, though, Kay showed that his own feelings were mixed. He wrote, "As I told you before you are

still in love with 'Dr. Black.' What you have accomplished
and what you are around the medical college and hospital has
created a glamour in which you are now basking. There have
been times when I wanted to hold you in my arms and kiss
you but invariably some little thing was said or done which
caused 'Elinor' to fade and 'Dr. Black' to appear. There were
times when I thought you did it deliberately... be careful that
you don't lose 'Elinor' she is of more importance."[9]

It was Kay who lost Elinor. Several of Elinor's Winnipeg
friends later recalled the relationship, and two of them
thought Elinor and Orville had actually been engaged for
awhile. But none of the factors that had challenged Elinor's
previous romance had really changed. Prior to Orville Kay's
letter, Elinor had received an adoring letter from a woman in
England. Kay was probably right when he sensed that Elinor
was deliberately evoking "Dr. Black" to avoid intimacy with
him. Elinor was still sorting this issue out. Furthermore, like
Bernard, Kay was made uneasy by Elinor's professional life.
One of the feminist writers on Elinor's bookshelf had an
interesting angle on this problem, citing "the need of men in
the complicated modern scene of women whose nerves are
not disturbed as their own are by the competitive struggle."[10]

Elinor was definitely in the thick of the competitive
struggle, with all the "clang and clamour" and "traffic of rude
voices" that Charlotte's offering to Elinor's teen autograph
book had warned about. Far from basking in glamour, Elinor
was having her nerves disturbed regularly at the General and
she wrote Charlotte about it:

April 29, 1939
My dear Larley,
    ... Tomorrow I finish on the Ward. I think the month must have
strengthened my character considerably if nothing else.
    Boy! what a little spasm of hell chucked into a lifetime!
    However I have maintained my dignity and said nowt, and have

got in some swell licks at operating on me own (more ways than one because the Senior interne has been a deliberate obstructionist instead of an assistant at the ops. You mind the long story I told you about him and the Caesars? Well he has been worse than that but I won't bore you with the details.) ... I'm not resigning; I'm sticking around until I'm fired — Isabel Mc says it is much better for the character.[11]

Along with this update, Elinor sent Charlotte some money, ordering her to "damn well accept [it] *graciously*" because Elinor was sending it as a votive offering to the gods — patient's collections that month had been the best yet.

Holding one's own at the General was hard at times; many women doctors agreed on that, recalling various attempts to discourage or humilate them. One woman said she was told it wasn't worth it to apply for a residency because no one would ever go to a woman specialist in private practice. She was also told that some people *would* go, but they'd be male exibitionists. Another woman, an anaesthetist, had the experience of being dismissed, in front of a patient, by a doctor who "did not let women work for him." The surgeon interrupted her explanation to the patient with, "Thank you very much. Dr. So & So will give my anaesthetic." Many years later, there was still pain in the words, "So there was nothing to do but leave, you see."[12]

These women, and others like them, had the impression that such incidents were aimed at eliminating them from the competition for patients. As one young woman heard from her father in 1859, "I agree to *all* you say in favour of working, — it is very honorable, very right and worthy of all praise, but what I object to is your taking money for it."[13] This message, unchanged in 80 years, lay beneath whatever patronizing or disheartening words were actually spoken. Elinor survived, one friend said, because she "could stare down anybody" and "never let down her professional guard."[14] That could be exhausting, as Elinor's letter to Charlotte showed. The growing practice meant more than money — it also meant validation.

Elinor's usual source of validation — D.S. MacKay — had suffered a serious heart attack. Within two years, he was gone. Elinor was also struggling with other losses. It hadn't worked out with Orville Kay, and Bernard had just written her, "Also I acquired a wife last summer which I can't remember if I have told you about or not?"[15] Elinor brushed this off when she wrote Charlotte about it, saying, "Well, I'm glad I aren't the one who was acquired so casually."[16]

In her next letter to her sister, though, Elinor wrote, "The more I think of you not coming to Winnipeg the more depressed I become; it is so kinda pointless trying to make oneself comfortable just for oneself, & yet there is no one in Winnipeg that I want to make comfortable too."[17]

Comfortable didn't seem to be a word Elinor could apply anywhere outside her own office. She was made uncomfortable at the hospital, she made Orville uncomfortable in their relationship and, as for the current Black family dynamics, even at a distance they made Elinor more than uncomfortable; they made her furious.

Margaret was showing signs of mental illness. She'd never been easy to live with, but now she was becoming increasingly difficult — she was starting to do things like give someone a present and then accuse the person of stealing it. Elinor was worried that Charlotte was going to take on too much of this. Elinor reacted — possibly to the fear that more losses were imminent — by blasting everyone. She wrote Charlotte, "Mother won't die: her type never do; she will hang on and on. . . . [Father] no doubt is getting quite a lot of balm to his soul out of being martyred. . . it is a good reaction for him after all the years that poor dear Daddy was so busy at the office that he never knew what was going on at home. As for Marjorie: she has managed to successfully bugger up almost everything that you have planned to do to date, and if you let her bugger this up too, you are a bigger sap nor I thought."

By "this" Elinor meant Charlotte's vacation. It sounds like Elinor could have used one as well. She pointed out, needlessly, that she was bad-tempered these days. She said a doctor would likely tell her to get more rest and better and more regular meals, adding — "yeah, that's why I don't go to see one."[18]

She worked instead. When not lecturing at the College, working at the hospital or seeing her own patients, she volunteered with St. John's Ambulance, teaching first aid and being present at large public gatherings to help if needed.

In May 1939, the king and queen of England visited Winnipeg and, as Elinor put it, "had everyone on their ears"[19] with excitement. In honour of this visit, Elinor was issued a new St. John's Ambulance uniform — a charcoal-grey suit and a hat with a red stripe denoting "doctor." Elinor found this amusing, telling Charlotte, "After me getting my 'Army' uniform, we aren't going to be inspected by them. I'm supposed to put it on and mill about rendering first aid: one look at the hat and the crowd will open a path of amazement for me."[20] Four months later, England and Canada were at war with Germany, and the uniforms were real. It would be years before Elinor, or any other doctor, could dream of getting "more rest."

A certain number of doctors and scientists were needed in Canada and not allowed to enlist (much to the intense frustration of some of them — one woman recalled being reminded of her status by a Mountie after she tried to sign up anyway). The burden on those who stayed home became increasingly heavy. Especially the teaching. The pressure was on to produce a lot of doctors quickly — Elinor called it "the diarrhoea curriculum" when two classes of students graduated in a single year. For the lectures she prepared and gave all year, Elinor was paid $109.24.

In this situation interns and residents were forced into more responsibility than they would normally have been given, and some of them leaned heavily on Elinor for help. And she had to make a living! Only through running her office could she bring in any money. Shortly before the war started, Elinor had happily bought a set of golf clubs but between exercise and sleep there was no contest and she soon gave up the game.

Elinor wrote briefly about this period but she didn't comment on whether or not the exhausting work was a relief from all her other worries. That she had plenty of other worries is evident from her papers. Charlotte wrote in November, 1940:

> Hellzapoppin around home too. For a week Mother has been possessed of a series of demons [Margaret was ramming around the house, constantly up and down stairs, reading at people]; . . . we got a new maid last Friday and Mother has been doing the mistress-in-her-own-home act for her. . . . Something has to be done with Mother — Dr. Wilson says increase her dope. . . . We will probably have to put her in an institution — it is either her or the rest of us; . . . don't you dream of coming home at Christmas for it is Hell! Zizzling love — Charlotte."[21]

Frank had written Elinor earlier about this family crisis, saying, "Charlotte and Marjorie will go forth to survey another 'Home' for Mother to-morrow. . . . She seems to be taking some interest in her fellows but was 'bouncing' according to the girls' report, last Sunday — which means hard to hold down and offering no immediate hope of her being able to return to the quiet life."

Frank didn't lose the opportunity of this letter to remind Elinor what life, in his view, should be about. He commented that a biography Elinor had sent him nearly merited the title "Great" but fell short: "If it had been the story about a 'Quest,' or of something to be achieved, it would have been so; but in effect it is but the struggle upwards of a youth, better endowed with brains than most of us; . . . at the end one is sorry that he had not been caught up with the divine afflatus in respect of some worthy cause."[22] He told Elinor to take care on the "assembly-line" her job had become.

Margaret was put in a "home." She wrote pleas to family members to be released, reminding them that she'd been a "good wife" and was now a "Forsaken Mother." On February 18, 1941, Frank wrote Elinor a bit about this, also telling her that coffee was really a very dangerous drug and that he must get after his income tax "for conscience sake, not for the money in it." He signed it, "With love and best wishes, Your Father, F.M. Black."[23] A few hours later, his heart gave out and he died.

The day after his death the *Winnipeg Free Press* reminded readers of the "great qualities of character and integrity that marked Mr. Black's whole career," and recalled him as a man "who carried the sternness of his convictions fully into his daily life. His standards were high and he maintained them at whatever cost. . . . His code was rigid and unbending but it was tempered always by a deep kindliness. . . . He will be remembered as a figure of great worth." Premier Bracken told the *Winnipeg Tribune* that Frank "shirked no task, no matter how unpopular, if he felt it was in the interest of the province." Bracken added, "I cannot speak too highly of him as a man and a citizen." A *Tribune* editorial said that Frank served the West for half a century — "Wherever there was need of a public-spirited man with administrative ability, integrity and the solid grounding of finance, there Mr. Black was called."[24]

Several weeks later, Frank's mother, the grandmother

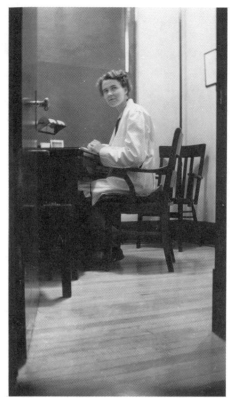

Dr. Black in her office, 616 Medical Arts
Building, 1941

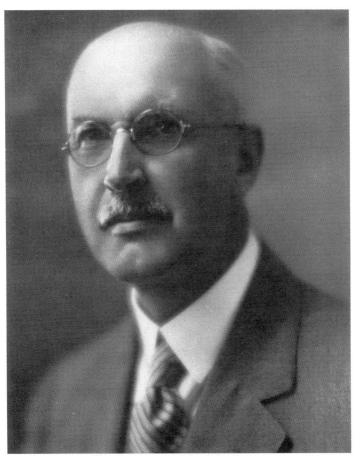

Frank Black (Department of Archives and Special Collections, University of Manitoba)

Elinor had spent her seventh year getting to know, wrote her, saying, "I loved his bright cheerful letters and now feel that he is no where on earth." Elinor was 36. For more than half her life she'd measured her achievements and thrown her stubborness against the man who signed letters, "Your Father." Now she was truly on her own.

Her grandmother's letter reinforced this realization and it also underlined Elinor's worry — and cause for worry — about her friends and relatives in Britain. Mrs. Black wrote, "All the dreadful happenings make me very miserable. Surely it cannot be much worse now and God in his might may yet help & save — let us not lose hope, and Hitler be overthrown, tho he has all the powers of Evil helping him."[25]

Annie French Rhead also hoped Hitler would be overthrown — by the measles. In spite of air-raids and bombs — her house was severely damaged by blasts from near misses and the beloved conservatory fell to rubble — measles was the worst fate Rhead could bring herself to wish on anybody. Through coal shortages, explosions, warnings from the government, a condemned notice tacked to her door and pleas from her brother, Rhead stayed put. Perhaps she felt it was unfair to abandon the fairies, surely the most innocent of all the victims of the Blitz.

Another friend in England wrote to Elinor about the bombing. With cheery aplomb, her friend described this incident at her home in Kent: "We've had two doses of incendiary bombs in our back & front gardens! The 2nd time I was alone. . . . I saw one on our front fence! gave it 2 mins to explode! advanced cautiously with sandbag, lifted high to protect face! suddenly 2 enormous HE's [Heinkel bombers] whizzed over! down I flopped under the shrubs! giggled a bit! rose! restored sandbag technique! advanced & covered bomb!"[26]

The South London Hospital for Women, and Elinor's

friends and colleagues there, were dramatically affected by the bombing. South London's location was such that close-by bombing was inevitable, and a special act of Parliament overruled the hospital's charter so that male patients could be treated there. As Margaret Louden, Elinor's former supervisor, recalled, "It would have been impossible to sort the women from the men during each major influx of serious casualties. Sometimes we would put up half a dozen blood transfusions within minutes of the casualties arriving, and to have sent the men on elsewhere would undoubtedly have cost lives." (The hospital reverted to its charter as soon as the war ended.)[27]

South London was designated a casualty hospital, and the Outpatient Department Elinor had worked in was now the Casualty Reception Ward. A troop of Rover Scouts pitched in to help the depleted medical staff by working as orderlies, messengers, stretcher-bearers and fire-watchers. Bombs dropped in the hospital gardens, in neighbouring roads; the hospital's new nurses' home sustained a direct hit.

Elinor battled her way through 1941, the crushing work, the grief at the loss, in different ways, of both her father and her mother, the worry for so many friends in England, the loneliness. She battled on, but as the year ended she made a startling discovery — someone had finally broken through *her* defenses. She was in love, and so was he, and Elinor was suddenly coping with an entirely different kind of problem. Her lover was married.

The evidence of this love affair is filed away in one of the most fascinating folders among the thousands of pieces of paper Elinor left behind. Elinor went to great lengths to clarify and organize her papers but this file, neatly labelled "Boyfriends" raises more questions than it answers. Bernard's letters are in there, so are Orville Kay's. There's also a stack from a man Elinor considered a silly nuisance who couldn't take a hint if it was slammed down in his ear. Repeatedly hung up on, this poor fellow resorted to letters, where he insisted that he would rather die a thousand painful deaths than inconvenience or irritate Elinor for one second so if she would only find it within her to drop one word — just one word — such as "sick" or "busy" in an envelope and send it to him, he would understand completely and never again — and so forth. He almost drove Elinor mad. And yet, one of these letters, seemingly indistinguishable from the rest, was carefully typed up by Elinor with this note on the bottom in her handwriting: "All the inked mistakes are the ones he made & are corrected as he corrected them. The occasional wrong key in the typing are my 'hurrying mistakes.'" Elinor was a poor typist but she was an archivist *extraordinaire.*

It appears that with this particular letter Elinor did the typing and notation upon receipt. That would indicate that the boyfriend file was already in place, not something she organized toward the end of her life. In another instance, Elinor made a copy of one of her replies to an admirer and put it, along with the gentlemen's two letters, in the boyfriend file. She did that only once, but the insouciant, flirtatious, and utterly woman-of-the-world tone she affected for her answer probably pleased her so much she was moved to make a copy. Most interesting of all is this: few people sign love letters with their full names, so Elinor thoughtfully provided these, in block capitals, under their signatures.

Did she fear that memory might fail her when it came time to write her memoirs? Or was she so sure, even as a young woman, that her papers would end up in the hands of an archivist or a biographer? And what were Elinor's criteria for inclusion in the file? She had many close male friends over the years and she kept all their correspondence too, but each of those men had either his own file or was put under "doctor friends." The boyfriend file is a mystery, and the feeling exists that some of the men in it — represented by no more than a single letter or a faded newspaper clipping — might be astonished to learn they'd been included.

Twelve men in all. But, from the available evidence, only one who truly mattered. There was one man who provoked a response, who didn't retreat in confusion when "Elinor" abruptly shifted into the cool and collected "Dr. Black." Getting past the superficial and down to the essence of things was his life's work. There are doctors, lawyers and soldiers in Elinor's boyfriend file — but the one who won her heart was an educator, an activist, some said a radical.

This man's letters sparkle with clear intelligence and challenge and passion. They tell the story of an old friend, passing through town, the usual social call shoehorned into two busy schedules, the usual exchange of news and camaraderie and admiration. But this time the words, glowing and tumbling in the space between them, trickled away. A bit shocked, their eyes met and they perceived each other as different from the way each had been just moments before. And once this was seen, it couldn't be unseen.

Later, he tried to remember, he fought sleep to remember exactly how it had come about, exactly how things changed, but it was now lost in a blur of happiness and disbelief that it could be true. He wrote about being carried away from her, in a train full of people who knew nothing of the waves of emotion flooding through him, and how impossible *that* was to believe, too. How could they not know? He wrote straight into his feelings — the quiet, rich radiance giving way to overpowering loneliness replaced in turn by an exultant desire to laugh out loud because it wasn't a dream.

Deep and abidingly you have come unto me.

Reality set in soon enough. He teased Elinor about the *careful* letters she sent to his office, but he admitted he shared her reservations about writing at all. He wrote her about running into a mutual friend who asked of news of her and how he struggled not to appear too enthusiastic or well-informed in his answer. He described his feeling of helplessness; he felt her anguish about the war and he knew if he were there he might save her at least some of the pain, alleviate the type of suffering that just turns round on itself, uselessly, and allows no healing. But he could rarely be there.

He felt her anguish too, over their situation. When Elinor used the term "poacher's rights," he understood the distress behind the flip remark. He didn't let her get away with words like that, he made a case for the right to joy, to moments in life that are beautiful and thrilling. He made a good case, writing lyrical, romantic and moving passages. Once he described walking the streets alone, entering a movie theatre and finding, in Joan Fontaine, an outline or a characteristic that reminded him of her, Elinor, and that comforted and cheered him. When he left the theatre, he wrote, he no longer felt alone.

When Elinor tried to project "Dr. Black" he didn't let her get away with that either. He respected her work, he referred to it often, he even looked up her article in the *Canadian Medical Association Journal* and tried to puzzle through it. He found it intriguing that Elinor could appear quite removed and distant when she was sitting a few feet away. Intriguing, not threatening — when she explained she had, of necessity, cultivated that quality, he understood. He just didn't want it used on him.

As 1942 ended, and through the following year, the letters focussed more and more on politics. He saw two kinds of people — those who felt the war was a people's war for real justice, and those who considered it a disturbance of a previously comfortable existence.

He started contributing to the Co-operative Commonwealth Federation (CCF), saying the development of the party would be counted as significant in Canadian history, saying people had to take the gamble, saying methods of education in times of crisis might need to become faster and more direct, saying Stan Knowles and Tommy Douglas were making an honest attempt to improve things.

He didn't see the same attempt — to improve things — being made in the church, and he feared the SCM was being co-opted to the point where kids who were "alive" no longer went near it. There were those in the SCM who believed real religious activity meant fighting for social change first, prayers after, and there were those who were afraid the SCM was losing the financial and structural support of the church and the important thing was to keep that relationship sound. These points of view seemingly could not be reconciled. It was the time of the Big Rows, and the word *communist* became an epithet.

People who had worked together for years were bitterly divided. Many must have felt as Elinor's lover did when he wrote and asked her if she knew what it was like to have people you cared about fail, utterly, to understand a critically important point.

Church politics, the CCF, Quebec (he wondered how Quebec could possibly learn that its fortunes were bound up with rest of the world if English Canada alternated between placating Quebec and threatening it), these issues gradually replaced the references to Joan Fontaine. By 1944, the romance had run its course. He sent her a sad little poem about being quite himself again.

Interestingly, while he was not himself, but rather still caught up in the altered state known as "in love," Elinor had sent *him* a whole book, a book by Winifred Holtby, saying this author "almost" expressed her. Interesting for two reasons: first, Holtby wrote passionately about feminism and work, saying that work was "the instrument to give you the power you need to work for the things you care about and fulfil your destiny and yourself. That is the only security and the only happiness."[28] Second, Holtby's personal life was devoted to passionate friendships with women, most notably Vera Brittain. Brittain and Holtby continued to live together after Brittain's marriage; the story of this intense relationship is celebrated in Brittain's book, *Testament of Friendship*. Whatever Elinor meant by "almost," sending Holtby's work to the man she was in love with was certainly also sending a message about who she — Elinor — was.

Elinor, according to other letters that start appearing in 1944, was deeply committed to her own passionate friendship with Gertrude Rutherford. So much so that Elinor risked a bitter break with her sister Charlotte over the relationship. Sadly, it's impossible to reconstruct the early years of this tremendous friendship (Elinor dated it, on various occasions, back to 1923) because Elinor — for reasons that will be discussed later — destroyed all but one of Gertrude's letters. It is possible, though, to know some of what happened in 1944-45.

In December 1944 Gertrude came to spend Christmas with Elinor. Gertrude had recently been on a tour of western Canada, calling, as usual, on the United Church to encourage the full participation of women. She stressed that young women "richly endowed and of superior capacity, must be drawn into the work, and a high standard of training must be demanded of them."[29] For over 10 years, as principal of the United Church Training School (dubbed "the Angel Factory") in Toronto, Gertrude had directed that training. She felt that the scripture "To him that hath shall be given" could be interpreted as "To him that hath the spirit, the will, the insight, and the capacity, will be entrusted the great responsibilities of the day." Gertrude lived her own life that way. But what she discovered on the Christmas holiday put an end to the great responsibilities she had thrived on.

Elinor had sent Gertrude to a specialist for a thorough check-up. Gertrude was only 51, but she hadn't been well, and there was a family history of heart trouble. Elinor was forwarded the devastating report — "Fluoroscopic examination of the chest showed greatly enlarged heart with the apex about one inch inside the lateral wall of the chest, and a bulging in the posterior cardiac space. The electrocardiogram is enclosed."[30] Gertrude could suffer complete heart failure at any time.

The shocked reaction of some of Gertrude's close colleagues in the church was swift. One wrote, "It isn't true, is it — and yet, I know it is or what caused the deepened furrows around her mouth and eyes but sheer apprehension of what the future holds for her. . . . I just can't imagine the Boss spending half her time in bed or on it and the other half in fear and trembling of doing too much." This same friend wrote again a few days later to say, "Though I did understand from the Boss and everyone else that she had been dealt a cruel smack, your letter nearly knocked me out! It looks so much worse in black and white, ye ken."[31]

One can only guess, from the hundreds of loving letters Elinor wrote to Gertrude over the next several years, just how terrible that specialist's report, in black and white, must have looked. One thing is clear — from that point on, Elinor's devotion to her friend's well-being became absolute, devotion that bordered on extreme possessiveness.

Devotion won out, however, when it came to Gertrude's marriage. In spite of her jealousy and dislike of Gertrude's choice — Murray Brooks, a colleague in the SCM — Elinor actively encouraged the marriage, talking to Murray about how time was short, shopping with Gertrude for the trousseau and even helping to pick out the ring. The wedding was set for December 6, 1945. Elinor's determination to be with

Gertrude as much as possible beforehand caused her to override previous plans with Charlotte. The way Elinor went about it caused Charlotte to explode in hurt and anger. A series of letters followed:

April 15, 1945
CHARLOTTE. I am feeling better physically and mentally I think. The thing that took my spirit was to realize that you had said to yourself I've got to go to Vancouver no matter how busy I am so it will be O.K. for me not to be in Winnipeg when Charlotte comes this summer.

Undated
ELINOR. I am still picking up my teeth from the various corners to which your slash on the jaw sent them. I wish that you had been frank to my face about your true feelings concerning my summer plans & my visit to you. As to the motives of that visit you seem to have them fixed in your mind to your own satisfaction and it is useless for me to argue the point with you. . . .
     I am sorry if I irk you & if you want to consign me to hell, I wish you would and get it over with. I have always been very happy in the friendship that we have had along with being sisters. I like you and your spasms of damn fool nonsense, what is *more* — I am proud to be your sister! . . .Let's not be cross with each other — it is silly, when we have always had such fun together; . . . seems funny to be writing you a letter in a more or less formal tone: this is the first and last I hope!

April 29, 1945
CHARLOTTE. What was the belly-blow about your recent visit was not learning that you will not be in Winnipeg if I go down in August — (after all when I wrote last fall that the convention was to be held I asked if I might use your apartment if that was the time you would be away) but the fact that you felt you had to lead up to telling me with an hour long story in justification. . . . You are wrong if you think you irk me — I enjoy your company more than that of anyone else. . . . Now let bygones be bygones.

May 5, 1945

ELINOR. Dear Perfessor,

Look, ya Lug, ya can't let bygones be bygones that way: that is kid's stuff, or like your Mother who never faced a fact from the front in her life; it is just a euphemistic way of putting a skeleton in a cupboard to let it go stomping about nights, or of burying a hatchet with the blade sticking out to cut your feet every time you go near the spot. That line ain't good enough, and if you have a peeve, I wish you would come out with it, and then we would both feel better. If it is the friendship between Gertrude and me that is sticking in your crop, you'd better get on with the job of swallowing it, and assimilating it, because you are going to have to take a lot of it and you might as well get used to it.

Shure — if you want to put it that way — I got an awful crush on her — bin crazy about her for 22 years, and look to be getting worse all the time, and that is saying something considering the usual mutability of my affections in past years. Anyway she is the best friend I ever had, and the only person I know who can slap me down every time I open my mouth on any given subject — and it amazes me that she not only seems fond of me, but seems to respect my judgement in some things too. Well, now it looks like the rest of the chapters of her life are to be edited in an abridged edition. This I find very hard to take, and it is my intention to see as much of her in the next years as she and her husband and my job and geography will allow — and if you as my favorite sister can't see the sense in that, well — I'll be disappointed in you, that's what — But maybe this hasn't been bothering you at all, but you kinda acted like it was, and if I am on the wrong scent — well, you can skip the above having filed away my feelings on the subject for future use and reference.

That was clear enough. Elinor was not about to brook any interference in her time with Gertrude and insinuations about having an "awful crush" on her friend would be met with defiance and pride. Charlotte's final letter on the subject was subdued, sad and perceptive. She realized where her hurt truly lay: "I don't think jealousy bothers me because you have always had very good friends with whom you did things. You were always very generous in your time to me — you played tennis with me when it would have been much more

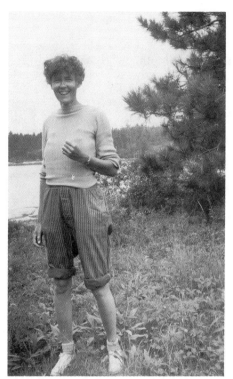

Elinor, French River, Ontario, 1943

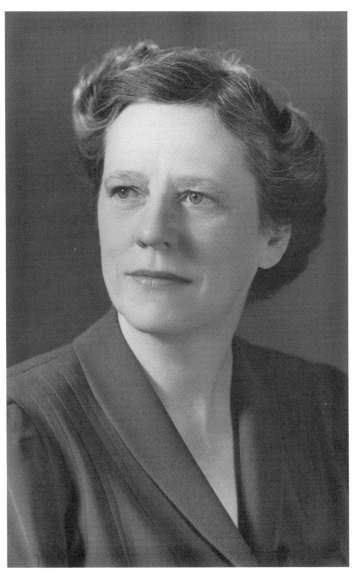

Gertrude

fun to play with others and so forth. The thing that sticks in my crop is that I have laughed and planned with you quick trips home so you would not have to spend your holidays there, and about Marjorie's visits with you in Winnipeg. Now I find myself "one of the family" and have to laugh on the other side of my face, which hurts."[32] Much as Elinor denied it, this had the ring of truth. Henceforth, Elinor *would* worry about spending "enough" time with Charlotte — enough to get away guilt-free to Gertrude. Charlotte knew it, and the two sisters would never really recapture their former closeness.

Another person Elinor was close to, and usually tried to see when she went east, bowed to Gertrude's larger claim — although a bit wistfully. She wrote, "Just because you adore Gertrude should not make you forget that I adore you. And I would dearly love the chance to show you off once in a while."[33] But she knew she wouldn't get that chance in the face of Gertrude's diagnosis, and she tried to comfort Elinor, not pressure her. She wrote, "I know how lost you are going to feel but friendship like yours does not ever end and look at all the years you subsisted on letters. You can do that again and — God help me — whether she is in this world or out of it, I don't really think it will make any difference to your feeling of beautiful security with her; she is going to be right there when you need her, no matter where she is. That relationship has gone on too long to let a little thing like marriage or death change it."

Elinor had seen too much death in the past few years — death and suffering and worry. D.S. MacKay and her father were gone. In one of his last letters, Bernard had talked of preparing to be called back into the Royal Navy; after 1942 he doesn't appear in the British Medical Association directory. In 1943, Donald was admitted to a sanatorium, fighting his second active bout of tuberculosis. TB was a killer. Donald was kept at the sanatorium for 15 months (Elinor sent her eldest sister Marjorie the money for Donald's medical bills, instructing her that Donald was not to be told where the money came from.) By 1944, Elinor's plucky friend in Kent, who once giggled while covering bombs, could only write grimly, "So jolly to hear Churchill promise us that the hardest fighting is yet to come."[34]

Tragedy struck close to home. Throughout the 1930s Elinor had become increasingly close to the Pickersgill family. She and Jack, who would one day be described as "the political manager of the Liberal Government,"[35] enjoyed theatre and arguments. Jack loved to get Elinor's goat by suggesting that medicare was a good thing because, for example, if he had to spend 20 percent of his time billing students he wouldn't be as competent a lecturer in history, would he? Logically, then . . . and so forth. Elinor categorically rejected the comparison. Elinor and Jack and Bessie and her twin brother, Walter, socialized as a gang, and Elinor loved their home, so different from the austere one she had grown up in. She sometimes told her friends, "You Pickersgills are so smart to have picked your mother."[36] Frank was another Pickersgill brother, a younger member of that lively household. By May 1945, Elinor knew that Frank had been executed at Buchenwald.

Elinor shared that sorrow. She also saw her relationship with her lover end, and of course the friendship they'd had was forever changed. So was Elinor's friendship with Charlotte. And Gertrude, the woman Elinor had "bin crazy about for 22 years and look to be getting worse all the time," was facing an "abridged edition" of life. Then, in 1946, Elinor's mother died. The stiff coolness that had existed for years between Margaret and her last-born was never resolved.

And all the time Elinor was coping with one upheaval after another in her private life, there was the continual struggle against another kind of loss in her public life — her identity as female, her sense of self as a woman.

In 1944 a Vancouver paper ran an article called "Successful in Man's World." The article set out to debunk "the theory one must be strictly masculine and slightly peculiar" to succeed and profiled four local women who had. Charlotte (whose large photo topped the article) was one of the four; she was a professor in the University of British Columbia's Department of Home Economics. The newspaper also did columns on an engineer who was also an "A1 cook," a law student who had been elected president of the Law Students' Society, and a doctor, described in the article as a "full-fledged 'medical man.'"[37]

Elinor too got her picture in the paper in the 1940s — a nice-sized photo in a panel of four. The first three panels showed three male colleagues; Elinor shared her panel with Dr. Gerda Flemming. The headline above them all read, "Canadian Medical Men Gather in Winnipeg."[38]

In Vancouver the successful woman doctor was a medical man, in Winnipeg Elinor was one of the medical men who gathered, and in a 1944 issue of the *Manitoba Medical Review* an ad for baby formula had a cartoon of a vigorous formula-fed baby crowing "My Doctor's Made a New Man Outta BOTH of Us!"[39]

Doctors were men, and women were — patients. In 1879, the Ontario College of Physicians and Surgeons exam discussed remedies for patients in labour exhibiting "wild tossing about, accompanied with petulance and irritability" or, conversely, "uterine inertia in a patient of mild, tearful disposition."[40]

In 1983, a medical-school textbook entitled *Obstetrics and Gynecology* carried a chapter, written by three men, called "Psychology and Life Periods of Women." The authors described how to evaluate a patient's personality: "It begins as she enters the consultation room and sits down. Character traits are expressed in her walk, her dress, her makeup, her responses to questions, and in almost every action, both verbal and nonverbal in nature. The observant physician can quickly make a judgment as to whether she is overcompliant, overdemanding, aggressive, passive, erotic, or infantile."[41]

Given that the attitude expressed in the 1879 exam was still present, even expanded upon, a hundred years later, it's unlikely Elinor failed to notice it. At what point did Elinor stop giving enthusiastic talks on the achievements of medical women and start saying, as some people remember her doing, "I don't get on with women"?

It's more that Elinor couldn't *identify* with women, if one defined "women" the way textbooks, *Canadian Home Journal* and *The Canadian Doctor* did. Elinor had cherished enviable friendships with many women, some of whom were as accomplished and successful as she was. She occasionally helped younger women who looked up to her as a "port in a storm" and a "compass" one could go by. A common reaction to this biography from Elinor's former obstetrical patients was, "Oh, I just *worshipped* Elinor Black."

Yet no one seemed to think it strange when Elinor said she didn't get on with women. Imagine the reaction a Canadian would provoke if he or she went around saying "I don't like Canadians and I can't get along with them." Perhaps her comment was accepted because of the way Elinor started to define women.

There is some evidence that Elinor couldn't get along with, for example, fluttery elderly ladies. One reported to the nephew who had referred her, "Dr. Black was rough. I just *couldn't* go back there."[42] Elinor was liable to be rather blunt with some patients — "I hear you're getting married. Are you a virgin?" Not every young woman in the 1940s appreciated this style of taking a medical history. One woman interviewed was resentful at the cold way Elinor treated her when she reached out for some comforting, or mothering, during her labour. She was later astonished that Elinor "would do such a human thing" as call her husband with the news of the birth.[43]

And Elinor definitely had ambivalent feelings about other women doctors. She helped some, and became friends with others, but, as she became more successful, she distanced herself from the Federation of Medical Women of Canada (although she paid dues for years). In letters she sniped at some of her female colleagues, especially "the kind of woman doctor" who announced herself and took temperatures and pulses of people who felt faint on buses.[44]

The above "types," along with the wives in the *Canadian Home Journal* advertisement whose *husbands*, if they were modern husbands, answered the doctor's questions about the pregnancy and received the medical information, represented "women" to Elinor. And what was she? "Just a doctor." Elinor had always survived, and even thrived, by being one of the boys, a medical man like them. Being a medical man carried a lot of privileges and Elinor had worked long and hard to share in them. Some of the boys tended to think in terms of "us" and "them," the way they had in the "Say Men" article. Elinor definitely didn't want to be in the "them" category; she wanted to stay where she was, or even better, keep rising.

Elinor could be a medical man but she couldn't, obviously, be a male doctor. She could, however, be "just a doctor." Not a doctor and a woman, not a doctor who was, in fact, a woman — "just a doctor." This loss, of self, happened alongside all the other losses, but it was one Elinor never grieved, never even acknowledged. There was no time, in Elinor's life, for introspection. There was so much happening in her field, so much excitement. Medicine could expand to fill both sides of her. She asked for "no other blessedness"; she had "a work, a life purpose." She was publishing, she was considering entering the baffling and fascinating new field of endocrinology, she was planning a world tour of obstetrical centres. And, like every other GP and obstetrician in North America, she was up to her ears in the baby boom.

Seven

THE MATERNITY PAVILION:
"Safeguarding Motherhood"
▼

*Many wonder . . . what you are going to do after your re-
turn, whether you are going to do only endocrinology. . . .
You've got 'em guessing, boss. . . . There is still much curiosity as to who will be the next prof. in O&G.
(Letter to Elinor)*

THERE WAS, Dr. Fred McGuinness decreed, to be a new
maternity hospital in Winnipeg. In view of the terrible
epidemic of childbed fever in 1936, this new hospital would
be separated from the General, except for a connecting
tunnel. To further reduce the risk of any introduction of
infection, there would be no gynaecology cases admitted.
This would be maternity only, the Maternity Pavilion,
McGuinness' exclusive project.

F.G. McGuinness, head of obstetrics at the General in the
1940s, liked to rule by decree. He was frequently described as
a "dictator," an "autocrat" and a "prima donna" who wasn't
much given to sharing his reasons or his information. But he
was widely given credit for fighting hard enough for the new

maternity hospital to make it happen. Elinor wrote that McGuinness "bulled" the hospital into existence "practically by individual effort."[1] Elinor admired the "bulling," but she resented not being consulted so much that she was still complaining about it — and criticizing everything about the Pavilion's design — 40 years after it was built. At the time though, she needed that hospital as desperately as any other obstetrician in Winnipeg. She pitched in where it counted — raising money.

In one of her fundraising efforts on behalf of the Pavilion, Elinor made a graph for "the big shots of the business world." She showed them how, at the General, 900 deliveries and 60 maternity beds in 1939 had become over 2,000 deliveries in 1947 — with no increase in beds. Elinor thought her graph was "something business men could understand and no fooling."[2] Some of these men had probably already heard all about it from their wives, and no fooling. One doctor called the post-war maternity wards at the General "the black hole of Calcutta."[3]

Elinor's official account of the period was more restrained. This is what she wrote in her history of the department:

> The hospitals could scarcely cope with the extra load imposed on their maternity wards. Beds were brought up from storage and put in the corridors, and patients, husbands, doctors and nursing staff grumbled. One's telephone would waken one during the night with the message that a multipara had gone into labour; speed in getting her to the hospital was of the essence. But where to send her? Most of us had favourite hospitals where at least a corridor bed could be found for our patients so one would telephone, say the General but be sadly yet politely told that there was no vacant bed, even in a hallway. One would try the St. Boniface and get the same answer, then the Grace to receive another negative. Then the Misericordia and finally the Victoria, where one's name might not even be recognized, but no bed was to be had anywhere. Nothing for it but to call the General again and explain to the admitting officer that no place

could be found in any other hospital and could they please put up just one more bed in a corridor? It usually worked, so the patient was notified and sent on her way. But that did not mean that one could go back to sleep free from concern, for one could remember that there were two or three other patients just at term and what if they were to phone? It was a time full of tensions.[4]

It certainly was, and part of that tension arose from the fact that doctors and admitting staff were considerably less polite than Elinor portrayed them here. One obstetrician said doctors ranted, screamed, begged and openly threatened the hospital. He recalled, "You couldn't get your patient in. *Nowhere.* It wasn't until it was truly dire that we got the patient in."[5]

Tempers had got short in the lab too. As early as 1944, Dr. Cameron of the Department of Biochemistry was complaining in print that there was a definite limit to the number of doe rabbits available for the Friedman pregnancy test, yet doctors were ordering over 70 tests a month. Cameron said that his technicians were kept too busy doing pregnancy tests to assist in the department's research work, and the test was being ordered, in far too many cases, just to relieve the patient's mind when "a delay of a few weeks [would] permit the usual clinical diagnosis."[6] Such cases constituted an abuse of the technology, in Cameron's view, and if the obstetricians didn't stop it, his department might be forced to discontinue the test. Obstetricians added lab facilities to their dream plans of the new Maternity Pavilion.

As for the real plans, Elinor wrote that a few houses near the General were demolished in 1946, machinery moved in to dig the excavation and then — nothing. The hole in the ground remained untouched for almost two years while rumours flew about quarrelling architects and piles driven in the wrong place.

In the meantime, happily, it wasn't all frayed nerves and

cramped conditions. The 1940s also brought the discovery of the Rh factor — the kind of discovery that makes everyone remember why medicine is more than hospital politics. The excitement was tremendous.

When Elinor was in medical school, "jaundice of the newborn" was a mysterious condition treated by giving the baby an injection of the mother's blood. As Elinor wrote, "That didn't do much good,"[7] and most of these babies, suffering from jaundice, anaemia and brain damage, died. By the early 1940s, Dr. Bruce Chown was doing work in Winnipeg on the Rh factor that later brought him international recognition. By 1944, Elinor and other obstetricians and general practitioners in Winnipeg were getting calls from Dr. Chown regarding Rh testing for pregnant women. Chown told his colleagues that he would test their patients for free if he could be present when those women who tested Rh-negative delivered their babies.[8] In 1945, Dr. Chown started doing replacement transfusions within hours of the delivery, and the technique was working. Dr. Harry Medovy, paediatrician and author of *A Vision Fulfilled*, a history of the Children's Hospital in Winnipeg, remembered it this way:

> Soon Dr. Chown and his staff were answering calls at all hours in delivery rooms at all of the city hospitals. . . . When the Rh service was extended as a Department of Health service to the entire province, the staff followed. They were exciting days. It meant going out at any time day or night, in all kinds of weather, not only to Winnipeg hospitals, but to rural hospitals miles away. Approximately 250 affected babies were seen each year; the babies saved providing the exhilaration; those who died (about 25%), the depression.[9]

The discovery of the Rh factor was a true breakthough, a story with a happy ending. Elinor undoubtedly took joy in this victory for paediatrics that affected some of her patients so directly. In her own field, the increasing use of natural hormones, and the development of synthetic ones, were being promoted as a similar boon. In 1944, a full-page ad in the *Manitoba Medical Review* advocated "sex hormone preparations" for delayed puberty, impotence, amenorrhea, dysmenorrhea, sterility in men or women, vaginitus, morning sickness, missed abortion, habitual abortion, induction of labour and — once conception had occurred and been maintained and babies finally born — as a lactation suppressant.[10]

Similar ads in 1945 pledged a better world for women through "gynesic pharmaceuticals." One ad suggested that *all* patients, "however severe or mild their symptoms," could benefit from natural estrogen preparations. Another, written in 1945, has the feeling of Huxley's *1984* — "Fortunately, today, medical provision of 'tranquillity' for climacteric ["change of life"] cases is more practicable than ever — with Hexital . . . a preparation assuring more complete control of psycho-physical disturbances through ample hormonal compensation and safe sedation."[11]

A medical article in 1944 suggested by its title that menopause was something needing to be "diagnosed" and "treated." The article stated that it was "well established that the sex hormones are specific therapy for the climacteric."[12]

Elinor wasn't so sure. She wrote often, and eventually scathingly, about the use of hormone replacement therapy as a "treatment" for menopause. But that didn't mean she felt hormones should never be used under any circumstances. Her first article on the subject of hormones, published in the *Canadian Medical Journal* in 1942, took a cautious look at the "increasing use of androgenic substances in gynaecological disorders."[13] She reported the results of her experiments with hormone treatments on women who suffered from a variety of problems including debilitating periods, irregular uterine bleeding and breast pain. In general, Elinor thought the treatments had been helpful. But she felt that the whole idea of hormone therapy was far from "well established," never mind a breakthrough for women.

She wrote that the main difficulty with hormone treatments was "the natural variability of the menses" and that variability was something yet to be understood. She stressed how every women's endocrine makeup was different, and endocrine inter-relationships were "not yet fully explored" either. She didn't think hormone treatments for pelvic inflammatory disease had been proven effective, and prescribing hormone therapy to a woman who was "spotting" was simply inexcusable. In her opinion, a diagnostic curettage was often sufficient. Elinor ended her article by saying that it was probably a good thing hormone treatments were so expensive — the cost prevented using them as "a casual form of therapy in the menopausal patient, too many of whom are unfortunately prescribed for without a pelvic examination being made."[14]

Her next article, "The Uses and Abuses of Endocrine Therapy," published in the *Manitoba Medical Review* in 1945, expanded on the themes she hammered home for years. She wrote, "Too many women in the fourth decade are labelled simply 'menopausal' by their physicians, given a prescription for some oestrogenic preparation, and dismissed without any or adequate examination." She wondered whether "one is justified in subjecting the female organism to onslaughts of potent preparations which may cause imbalance in other endocrine directions not yet understood." She felt that menstrual disorders should be looked at in terms of "improvement in general physique, relief of tensions and overwork, improved eating habits or a change in environment." She concluded with, "The literature put out by the pharmaceutical houses is natually enticing and glowing:

unfortunately it is from this source that some practitioners obtain what knowledge they have of endocrinology, and their patients suffer thereby. It is a physician's duty to attempt to understand the rationale of endocrine therapy before prescribing such treatment. Until definite patterns of reactions in the gonadal field are arrived at by trained investigators, hormonal therapy should be used cautiously and judiciously."[15]

Hormone treatments had their place, Elinor felt, sometimes, maybe, depending, but she just didn't like what she was seeing around her. She called it "abuse." Decades later, feminist health-care activists agreed with her. One of Elinor's former students described her attitude toward hormone treatments this way, "We'd better not [be] putting spanners in the works because we don't understand how the works work."[16]

Elinor wanted to understand; she was fascinated by endocrinology, calling it in 1945 a science "still in the early and confused stages . . . there is probably no other branch of Medicine which presents the same variability of opinion nor gives rise to so much controversy."[17] She thought that the field deserved great respect and she was eager for all the ramifications and inter-relationships to come clear. And why should paediatricians have all the fun? She decided to take a year, do a world tour of important obstetrical centres and see what she could learn.

She was finally ready to go by October, 1948. Several months before that, she had approached one of her former war-time students, someone she considered a protégé of hers, about taking over her practice. Dr. Otto Schmidt, fresh from his Membership exams in England, was delighted to start his professional life with the assistance of Elinor's car, apartment and large, established practice. It was not the last time Elinor did whatever she could to help a struggling student.

The Stoughtons had helped her when she felt desperate; over and over she balanced her moral books by helping young versions of herself.

Elinor started her tour in New York and saw the Stoughtons. She was shocked by the evidence of the hard times her patrons were facing. Some of the art objects were gone, presumably sold. The house was in bad shape. Pater, optimistic as ever, still went to the office every day, with lunch in a paper bag, but he was very elderly, and Elinor doubted strongly he had any work to do there.

Some months prior to this visit, Elinor had received an impulsive gift of $1,000 from an uncle in California. He sent similar cheques to all his nieces and nephews. Elinor had tried since receiving it to get her uncle to sign the cheque over to Pater, and finally, shortly before Elinor left New York, the cheque arrived. Elinor was visiting Donna when Pater arrived home, embarrassed about what his "Sweet Childe" had done now — and bearing a diamante pendant necklace from a Fifth Avenue jeweller to give to her. Elinor wrote that she choked up completely and almost wept — not from gratitude to her patrons-turned-paupers, who were giving some of her generosity back to her, but from sheer irritation and despair over the Stoughtons' beaming belief that tomorrow would take care of itself. Elinor left New York "feeling very unhappy" about them.[18]

By early in the new year her spirits had picked up. She wrote Jack Pickersgill, "Thanks for your Christmas greeting — but how can I come to Ottawa when I have taken a year's leave of absence to visit the "large Medical Centres"? You mean toss it in with New York, Phila[delphia], Baltimore, Washington, Duke University in Durham, N.C. & now Boston?! On the 22nd I am off to G.B. [Great Britain] & eventually Sweden. It is a great life."[19]

Away from the daily grind of teaching and practising,

Elinor was doing something she loved. It wasn't just the learning, it was having the time to observe and ponder and record. She kept a medical diary of her trip, describing the operations and grand rounds, the techniques and treatments. She sketched equipment and set-ups that interested her, and noted the fact that one hospital had "good quarters for doctors (male & female)." She applauded "exquisite surgery," but sneered at poor attitudes and language — doctors who "treated their subjects with a dangerous hey-nonny-nonny" or used terms like "rearable babies." Once, shocked, she reported one hospital's statistic that "twice as many babies die from birth injuries as people are killed in road accidents per year!!"[20]

Elinor made reference to the debate about "early ambulation." One doctor she met was against it, sticking to the idea that new mothers could start to "dangle" [their legs over the bed] on the fourth day, but not stand or walk until the tenth. Another doctor seemed to think that you got the mothers up on the second day or not until the tenth — nothing in-between.[21]

Elinor summed up the various debates in a few lines. She allowed her gift of observation greater play in the letters she wrote to Isabel McGill, her kindred spirit from the days at Annie McCall's hospital. Elinor had arrived to visit hospitals in Britain in January 1949, and by April she felt she needed some time off. She had a wonderful reunion with her friend, including a weekend in Dunoon with Isabel and another friend, Inspector Janet Gray, the first women inspector on the Glasgow police force. Elinor described the weekend in one of her short story/memoirs.

In "The Blue Grass Disaster," the three pals ambled into a chemist's shop where Elinor noticed an impressive pyramid of Blue Grass soaps and bath powders and bottles of toilet water. No sooner did she say, "Do you like this stuff?" and put her finger on the shelf than the whole thing crashed to the floor. The rest of the story is taken up with Elinor trying to pay for the damage (while mentally counting the traveller's cheques "safely around her waist") and Inspector Gray snapping into action denouncing the base of the display as unstable, and urging Elinor not to get in a "pack of cost trying to argy-bargy." Elinor was hustled out of there by her friends and into the nearest pub, where a poem, "The Song of the Wreckers," was duly composed to preserve the incident for posterity.[22]

That took care of that, as far as Janet and Isabel were concerned. But Elinor, who wrote the story decades after it happened, seemed to be trying still to make amends, explaining that she barely touched the shelf and that she really had tried to pay. Frank and Margaret's strict Presbyterianism had gone deep.

The connection between Elinor and Isabel had remained strong and this visit reinforced the bond. When Elinor left Scotland, she opened her heart to her friend in a series of letters, writing the first one from Oxford.

May 13, 1949
    My dear Pooh. . . . A slug has crawled into my beautiful spring-time garden: Gertrude has had, is having, or is about to have, a tonsil tag removed. It is awful stoopid to worry, but I do. Under local, of course, but that is no comfort. . . . Having spent the A.M. wandering among the Colleges & sitting on the bank of the Cherwell watching the lads & lasses punt past, I have had a *SWELL* idea: let's chuck everything & start all over again as undergraduates here — eh? We'd have to do it now in middle-age in order to get the most out of it; youth is so cluttered up with inexperience & preoccupations thereto attendant that I am sure it must miss all the best of the *really* important things. Let's, eh? . . . It is Sunday again, & I am lonely. There is no use pretending I am not. I have taken myself for a long walk in a sunny world washed overnight, I have written letters, I have read, I have washed Dunoon out of my hair, mended & sorted — & I am lonely. This day had to come — its hand was on my shoulder as we

sat on the front that last afternoon at Dunoon: the feeling is an old acquaintance that has to be met eye to eye every so often. . . . One might as well admit that persons who evoke an affectionate response retain a piece of one that is a poignant reminder for months to come that one cannot live to one's self alone. And as far as I know, there is no salve for the tender place except frank recognition & a thankfulness that an affectionate exchange has been made. . . . [Getting back on my medical schedule will mean that] once more I will just be the unemotional doctor that the bulk of my friends know; someway or another you have found a key that only 2 or three people know exists — so be it; but I must lock myself up again for ordinary world commerce from now on. . . .

Monday noon — Yesterday was well-lidded down by a neighbouring pianist playing Night & Day, Deep Night, Smoke g.i.y.e. & the whole gamut, except Chloe, as I went to sleep. Sort of a swan song to immaturity.

This morning your letter came — which I loved. I want to TALK to you. Oh *DAMN!!!* . . . My love, ever. Elinor[23]

Shortly after this letter, Elinor left England for Stockholm, where experiments were under way using radium capsules for uterine cancer. She continued to hold long conversations by letter with Isabel.

May 30/49 — S.S. *Britannia*
My dear Pooh,
 . . . Am at the Capt's table with a kindly Norwegian elderly couple on my left & an English Mr. Rutland on my right who does most amazing things with his eyebrows, nostrils, mouth, tongue & even tonsils (fine big throat he has) as he talks — can't look at him 'cause it makes my face work too.[24]

Elinor arrived in Stockholm on June 1, without a visa. She told Isabel that Cook's Agency hadn't mentioned the need of one, and her passport was "wrenched from her as twere her virtue."[25] One can well believe it, given Elinor's attitude to changing trains in Hitler's Germany. Authorities in Sweden prevailed this time, however, and after a morning in the police station, Elinor was allowed on her way with the proper visa and a stamp saying "kriminal" in her passport. Elinor had a love/hate relationship with travelling. In Sweden, the hate side was winning and she shared this experience with Isabel.

> June 1/49
> . . . I have been studying the 'phone book, map & dictinary for an hour: can't make anything of this language. . . . And another thing, I don't like this swaddling business they do with their bedclothes; I like to sleep all over the bed, not in a bundle. . . .
> I dunno why when I hit a strange place I get a hate of everything & just want to "coorie" down in a corner with all pseudopodia well drawn in & wait there until the 2 weeks or whatever are over & I can go back to someplace familiar.[26]

Elinor's hate of everything included hotel clerks who "tossed" her room key at her and waitresses with whom she fought "a war of attrition." But she couldn't win against "the ruddy town house clock strik[ing] every 1/4 hour 1, 1-2, 1-2-3, 1-2-3-4, as well as on the hour all night long." She was up anyway. The sky got light at 1:00 a.m., and her hot-water bottle had burst in bed. Elinor's mood in Sweden was such that the next time a clerk wouldn't look up from her desk, Elinor used her "North Dakotan hog-calling contest" voice.[27]

It got worse. Elinor's contact in Stockholm, at least from her point of view, was a man called Professor Kottmeier. Kottmeier, however, didn't seem too interested in this visitor from Canada. Elinor wrote Isabel, "I think he looks upon me as a nightmare from which he hopes to awake at any moment — though mind you, I'm trying not to be a nuisance." Kottmeier did take Elinor to the final session of a conference on radiology, where she listened to papers in Swedish for two hours and then attempted to mill about in a crowd where she knew no one. (Kottmeier had left her, saying simply "I go now.") After a half hour of this "uproariously good time" she spotted him across the room and "gambolled over to him looking all tail-waggish & he literally shuddered." Elinor decided to give up, told Kottmeier "I go now" and left.[28]

Elinor had been made unhappy at the radium clinic also. Not because of language problems or people ignoring her, but because of what she observed. She wrote Isabel:

June 4/49
    ... Now if you were here I could tell you all about how they use radium in the uterus, & believe me, it is something!! I don't wonder that they perforate them sometimes. But you know, Isabel, it is downright depressing: they have had this organized Ca [cancer] set-up here since 1914 & yet of the seven new cases this morning, 3 were very far advanced & 2 of those had been treated by doctors for 6 months for anemia & never a vaginal exam done. What's the use of teaching and propaganda?[29]

June 10/49
    ... When we get our Ca's of the corpus we won't come to the Rh [Radiumhemmett] to get treated. They tell me they perforate 10% of uteri with the intracavitary packing of the radium — well, they done 4 of them Sat. A.M. & they perforated 2. Musta bin a bad morning. So after making the hole, they pick up an elongated applicator from off the radium desk & they insert it into the uterus so all the bugs can flit gaily into the peritoneal cavity & wot the hell — she's gonna be put on penicillin anyway. ... I'm not impressed.[30]

With all the disappointments and stress of the trip, it's easy to imagine how overjoyed Elinor was to be invited to a luxurious dinner party of expatriate Canadians. All that homesickness and bottled-up conversation had a place to let loose, and there were "small world!" connections in every new introduction. Elinor described the dinner as a "C.B. de Mille spectacle," and evidently she found herself a role in it. The next day she wrote Isabel, "When I saw what was in the mirror this morning... it made me wonder if I really had been so Frightfully-my-dear-Bright at the party, but there was no use trying to recall."[31]

Elinor must have been glad to leave Sweden behind. Back in London, she continued to share her thoughts with Isabel. Now that Elinor was leaving for Canada, Gertrude was even more than usual on her mind. She wrote Isabel, "Gertrude reports herself well — she never wittingly misleads me, but I never know how she is until I see her: sometimes it makes my heart sob & sometimes it makes it sing — but always I am happy to be with her again."[32]

Elinor, in an introspective mood, went on: "And while I smoke a last cigarette I might as well tell you something about me that you'll find out sooner or later: I'm not an all happy & pleasant person; I'm cross, irritable, bad-tempered, hypercritical & hard to live with. I'm only pleasant when everything is the way *I* want it — & then I get tired of it & get c,i,b-t,h, & h-t-l-w all over again. That's why I live alone. And then I get tired of myself & have to have people, & then I get tired of people — & it's a vicious circle & I'm always in some phase of it." By the end of this letter Elinor felt she could "greet" (cry), and wrote, "You wouldn't believe how much I have wanted you here for a final visit."[33]

As soon as she was on board the ship, Elinor continued writing the conversation in her head that was connecting her to her friend.

> My dear Pooh, I'm not happy just setting here on this big boat & contemplating sharing the cabin with three strange women & I don't think it is fair that they aren't distributing mail until after we sail tomorrow . . . especially when you've had such a good time in a country & are kind of depressed leaving it anyway & especially depressed about leaving a friend you would like to have about 4,000 miles closer & all you can do is hope that the friend is missing you too & that maybe after a day or so your spirits will pick up a bit so you can write her a decent letter & not just a moan that is really meant to tell her that you love her very much & hope to see her at the first possible moment.[34]

Isabel felt the same way. Over the summer she had written Elinor, "There is a mist of enchantment descending over the roads we travelled and the places we visited. ... I can hear the click and see you opening your door and I didn't imagine it for you were really there." She also wrote, "Your dear, dear letters — so like you that I just don't believe you aren't around the corner and I'll see you presently. ... When your first letter came I wanted to 1) write at once; 2) catch a train; 3) grab a phone."[35]

Any letters Isabel sent to the ship to console her friend or keep up her end of the conversation would have been addressed to *Miss* E.F.E. Black. Elinor asked her to do this. It's not clear when she began the practice, but by 1949 Elinor did not identify herself as a doctor when she travelled. Unable, as Frank and Margaret's daughter, to *lie*, she evaded questions about what she did, or, if pressed, mumbled something about teaching biology. She told friends she did this so people wouldn't bore her with their medical problems. But she also described herself to Isabel as "the unemotional doctor" who "locked herself up" when she functioned as such. Elinor had by this point been struggling for 20 years to be recognized as "just a doctor." Partly she chose it, partly this attitude was forced on her. Forced because of the way women — patients and doctors — were treated in the environment where Elinor spent most of her time. The in-joke around the General was that Elinor was "the only doctor in the [obstetrics-gynaecology] department who wasn't an old woman." All the other doctors in the department were men. The medical students liked the joke, changing it to Elinor being the only doctor in her department with balls.

Elinor was used to ignoring half her identity. Free of work, in situations where nobody knew her, she denied the other half. It's as though she wasn't able to integrate the two selves, or, out of resentment, wouldn't do so in one place if she couldn't in the other.

It was only a few days of shipboard subterfuge and then Miss Black would be in the place she called "Home," the place she felt most free and whole and happy. She would be with Gertrude.

Elinor arrived at Brookscliffe, Murray and Gertrude's summer home in Mansonville, Quebec, on July 16. She continued her frequent letters to Isabel. Elinor wrote this in the first letter she sent after arriving: "I'm Home. I never get used to the terrific upsurge of thankfulness that fills my being whenever I find myself face to face with Gertrude again. There is a quality about that woman that gives me a sense of being transported into the security and peacefulness of Abraham's bosom & I just get all comfortable & happy. . . . When she dies it is going to be — well, quite a thing."[36]

Elinor kept an eye on Gertrude's stress level, and one day she noticed her friend was looking like she had "lost control of her world" and was "fixing to have a row with somebody." That night, Elinor took Gertrude out in the canoe and "needled her until the storm within her broke" [on Elinor's head]. Gertrude was then able "to look at the pieces & decide they weren't up to much" and go back to sitting "loose in the saddle."[37]

Elinor wasn't always able to sit loose in the saddle herself. Gertrude's husband, Murray, got on Elinor's nerves. He got on her nerves to the point that one of Gertrude's friends sent Elinor a note suggesting that Elinor take herself in hand and tolerate Murray "for Gertrude's sake; . . . you can do anything for Gertrude's sake."[38] Elinor tried, but some days she didn't come out of her own little guest cabin at all. She said she didn't feel well. This made a strong impression on Mary Harvey, the 19-year-old student helping out for the summer.

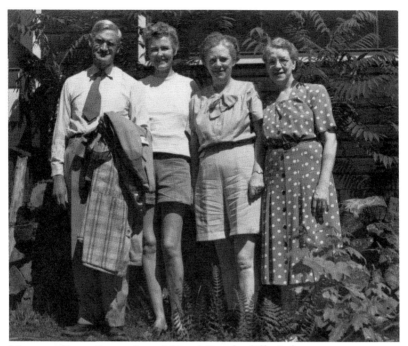

Murray, Elinor, Gertrude and friend: Brookscliffe, Lake
Memphramagog, 1950

It looked very much like sulking to her, and she had never seen an adult sulk like that.

Elinor made a great impression on Mary in general. Looking back on that summer, Mary recalled that she was a bit in awe of Elinor, never having met anyone like her before. Elinor was gorgeous *and* accomplished *and* physically strong and adept. Mary described Elinor as witty, bright, widely read and well-informed. No wonder Mary was anxious not to say or do anything stupid around her.

She needn't have worried. Elinor liked Mary, summing her up as "solid head, heart and legs, . . . young & resourceful & a handy little gadget to have along."[39] Compared to the age and fragile health of Murray and Gertrude, Mary's youth and vigour refreshed Elinor. They went swimming together, sat on the dock and talked. Elinor shared a bit about the man she had loved. She taught Mary to drive, and made sure she wasn't too burdened down with housework. She helped the youngster, who was serious and conscientious, to see the funny side of things. Elinor was a good mimic, and to make Mary laugh she imitated the broad accent of a woman in England who had trotted along the train platform, calling to her daughter, "Write me when the baby can say ba-na-na." Once, when Mary accidentally dropped a dish rag in the setting Jello, Elinor whipped it out and said that no one would know the difference. They agreed not to tell Gertrude.

Elinor wrote Isabel, "Poor young Mary has come under my fatal spell."[40] That wouldn't have been surprising, if true. From her papers and from interviews, it's apparent that Elinor had that effect on several people. Home-movie footage of Elinor in her early forties show a beautiful, animated, vibrant woman. More than one good friend felt that Elinor's was "the larger personality in a bigger world"[41] and that the relationship was not one between equals. Some friends said they were surprised and flattered by Elinor's attention to them.

Elinor's relationship with Mary was like this, but it was a close and lasting bond nonetheless. Elinor paid for Mary's graduate studies in literature (again citing the Stoughtons as her reason), and took a keen and possessive interest in her progress. When Mary married and had children, Elinor loaned the family the money for a summer cottage, returning the loan payment each year suggesting the money go for the children's education. (Survivor of the Depression, Elinor always warned Mary that she might not be able to afford the gesture the following year.) The two women wrote back and forth the rest of Elinor's life, and it was to Mary that Elinor left her books and art collection.

Gertrude had played this sort of role for Elinor in the beginning, a larger personality, possibly a benefactor, certainly a role model. But this relationship had long since become one between equals and Elinor was "desolate" every summer when she had to leave the person she loved so much and who loved her. At the train station, Elinor sent Murray and Mary away and waited alone. The train was late, "it's always late," Elinor wrote Isabel, "God! how I hate to leave."[42]

Elinor wasn't back in Winnipeg "10 minutes" before she was asked to speak at luncheons and section meetings. She plunged back into teaching and practice, "42 patients already this month & the old ones pouring in." She wrote Isabel, "The more I think of the way I was working before I left the less I know how I did it," but she was soon working that way again.[43]

She was also soon irritated with McGuinness, as irritated as she had been before she left and for the same reasons. The outer structure of the Maternity Pavilion was now finished.

In her history of the department, Elinor wrote that McGuinness announced one day that the interior plans would be on display in the nursing office for one day from 9 to 11 a.m., "far too short a time for any of us to study the plans and too late for us to make any suggestions for alterations in what had already been done."[44] (A personal letter in Elinor's files indicates that while Elinor was away McGuinness did give some members of the department an opportunity to comment on the early plans.[45])

Elinor moaned to Isabel, "The new Mat. Pavilion is *awful*; ... laboring women are gonna have to be wheeled a city block from Labour Rooms to Delivery Rooms."[46] This was Elinor's favourite criticism, she used the phrase "wheeled a city block" repeatedly. If one measured from the first labour room to the farthest delivery room, it was true, it was a block, and doctors, nurses and patients would find the trip about half a block too long on many an occasion.

Elinor also complained to Gertrude:

> Gertrude, I want $10,000. Do you spose I could separate my sisters each from $3,000 of their patrimony? I want an X-ray machine for the new building so that every time we want a picture of a patient in labour we won't have to wheel her two city blocks & through the main floor of the power house with its furnaces & generators roaring like Hades. Freddie says it isn't necessary but the rest of us plus the X-ray men think it is. There's no money for it — & yet there are at least 121 toilets in the place in broad view. If I could raise me the 10,000 bucks, I'd put it in tomorrow — & be accused of buying myself into the headship.[47]

The headship was on Elinor's mind. When she wasn't irritated by the Pavilion, she was worried that McGuinness was running the department by remote control and no one knew what was going on. Elinor felt "more and more despair" about this, she said to a friend, and added, "Freddie shows no signs whatever of retiring."[48]

Elinor herself was gaining recognition. She was elected to the Faculty Executive, a precedent for a woman. Then she was elected a Fellow of the Royal College of Obstetricians and Gynaecologists. This was a bigger precedent. Elinor was the first Canadian woman to become a Fellow, just as she had been first to get her Membership. In addition to the Winnipeg papers, at least seven other newspapers across the country, and *Saturday Night* magazine, ran a photo and/or a story, most with the headline "Woman Doctor Named Fellow."[49] Elinor joined the listings in the *Canadian Who's Who*.

Congratulations on the Fellowship poured in. Elinor told some people that getting the Membership had meant more than receiving the Fellowship because the former had been achieved through hard work and examinations. But to Isabel she wrote, "Heh! Heh! I am awful thrilled, although I am pretending not to be."[50]

In the midst of this excitement, the Lord saw fit to play a trick on Elinor. That's the way she put it to Isabel, following up with this explanation:

> Ye mind Prof. and Mrs. Stoughton as I had hoped I had seen the last of in New York some 55 weeks ago? Well, blow me, if the Univ. of Manitoba has not seen fit to present him with an Honorary Ll.D., and he comes to Wpg next week, all jubilant to get it. The Architects are putting on a big show for him and among other things over that week-end is the Beaux Arts Ball. Prof. S. wrote me yesterday saying he would squire me to the Ball. Black has shure reached an all-time low when she gets took to a ball by an 86 year old non-dancing tee-totaller!! . . . He will probably catch his death of cold or have a heart attack, and there I will be. . . .[51]

Professor Stoughton did have a heart attack. And there Elinor was indeed arguing fiercely with a night porter who refused to let her in the no-women-allowed men's club where Pater was staying!

Pater had arrived two days previously, almost penniless

but full of excitement about the degree and the ball. He was disappointed Elinor had not dreamed up some artistic costume to wear. Elinor pressed $10 on him, although he insisted that five was enough. The next evening they went to the ball, where Pater had a great time, staying past midnight. At seven o'clock the following morning, he called Elinor, sounding frightened, about a dreadful pain in his chest. She rushed over, and, according to the Stoughton memoir, almost had to club the porter with her black bag before he would let her see Pater. Finally, the porter led her through the kitchen and up the back stairs. That way, Elinor wrote sarcastically, she "contaminated the Club as little as possible."[52]

Elinor took one look at Pater and called a cardiologist, who arrived quickly and ordered an ambulance. Pater was most worried about missing the two o'clock degree ceremony; Elinor was worried it would turn out to be a post-humous award. Pater was kept in the hospital for 12 days. He asked Elinor to pick up his things at the men's club. She was so reluctant to repeat what she called the "male-sanctum" experience that she thought of asking a man to do it. But she felt protective toward Pater's shabby possessions. She didn't want strangers to know how hard up he was. Packing his clothes, Elinor found his wallet. It had three American dollars in it — and the two fives Elinor had given him.

Settling Pater's expenses, dealing with his agitation about getting home, and getting him home alive had Elinor "fair daft with worry and responsibility"[53] but she managed all three. She wrote Isabel that she had had this idea that following her trip she might have "a nice quiet spell to put [her] house in order, but no."[54]

No is right. Elinor recovered from Pater's visit by the end of March. In late April, the Red River flowing through Winnipeg started to flood. Within days, the catastrophe was such that the army was put in charge of the situation. Large numbers of evacuees from the more flooded areas of the city were homeless. Army officials had to find places to put them and looking around they noticed the nice, new, dry, empty, almost finished Maternity Pavilion.

Eight

THE FLOOD!

▼

*We moved into this building on May the 6th, 1950
at the height of the Winnipeg flood. (Elinor Black to
Charles Templeton)*

*Isn't that rather an inconvenient time?
(Charles Templeton to Elinor Black)*

THINK OF A FROZEN RIVER IN THE WINTER. CONSIDER THAT, IN WINNIPEG IN 1881, THE CITY ENGINEER WANTED A SYSTEM TO MEASURE RIVER LEVELS. HE TOOK THE ELEVATION OF THE RED RIVER ICE THAT YEAR ON THE MAIN STREET BRIDGE PIER, MARKED IT DOWN AND CALLED THE POINT ZERO DATUM.[1]

IT IS EARLY SPRING, 1950. IMAGINE THE RED RISING, NOT SUDDENLY, BUT STEADILY, INEXORABLY, DAY AFTER DAY, WHILE IT RAINS AND RAINS. THE RIVER IS A SLOW ONE, MOVING ONLY A MILE AN HOUR — AT ITS "RAMPAGING" BEST, LESS THAN FOUR MILES AN HOUR. IT CAN'T GET OUT OF ITS OWN WAY. IT BECOMES A WALL, A LAKE, A *THING* THAT

LEANS AGAINST 30 MILES OF DYKES "WITH THE SEEDY AIM-
LESS AIR OF A DRUNK HANGING ONTO A LAMPPOST."[2] IT
LAPS OVER THE TOP, FINDS CRACKS, FORCES THE DYKES,
HERE AND HERE AND HERE, TO GIVE WAY. IN THE RED RIVER
VALLEY, 560 SQUARE MILES ARE UNDER WATER; IN WINNI-
PEG, SIX SQUARE MILES AND SPREADING. THE RIVER RISES TO
30.3 FEET ABOVE DATUM.[3]

On April 20, 1950, the *Morris Herald* reported that Harry
Shewman, member of the Legislative Assembly for Morris, a
farming community 45 kilometres south of Winnipeg, rose
in the House to call attention to the serious flood danger
facing residents in the Red River Valley. The minister of
Public Works replied that every possible precaution and
measures had been taken to "combat the menace and render
aid."[4] That may not have sounded that reassuring to Betty
Goosen, who with her husband, Walter, ran a farm outside
Morris. There had been a devastating flood just two years
earlier. This spring, Mrs. Goosen was nine months pregnant
and several miles from the Morris Hospital.

That same day, April 20, Elinor was sending reassuring
words of her own to Gertrude. Elinor was in a sunny mood, in
spite of having "one of those weeks where one just hangs
grimly in putting one foot in front of t'other . . . hoping it will
end sometime before something bursts." She was in good
spirits, even singing Good King Wencelas in response to two
inches of new snow, because she saw the mail truck "whoop-
ing along Ellice Avenue" and sensed Gertrude's letter to her
was in it. Indeed it was, and Elinor answered it right away,
mentioning, "The river has come up a lot more today, but I
don't think we will get it."[5]

Elinor's next letter to Gertrude, dated May 6, opened with
this unequivocal message: "We are in a State of Emergency."[6]

Between April 20 and May 6, Morris was "virtually washed from the map"[7] and the entire town evacuated, except for two Mounties, who stayed and used canoes to rescue people stranded in the top floors of farmhouses. One report had it that the Mounties canoed in and out of their own office.[8]

Mrs. Goosen had gone to the Morris Hospital on April 28, making the trip partially by boat. There, she hoped to wait out the remaining few days until her baby was born. But the flood workers couldn't save the Morris Hospital. When one of the last trains able to get through left Morris for Winnipeg on May 4, she was on it, expecting her labour pains to start any minute.

All the people on that train were heading into what flood accounts later called "Black Friday."[9] By May 5, the city gravel pits had turned out, in ten days, close to an average year's supply of sand and gravel.[10] Over 90,000 sandbags were filled and dragged into place. Volunteers tried to keep their spirits up by singing "If I'd-a Known You Was Comin' I'd-a Built a Dyke" and "Evacuate, It's Later Than You Think."[11] Tireless teenagers, described by one editor as "the purple-pants and bobby-sox set,"[12] exasperated their exhausted co-workers by spending their work breaks *jitterbugging* to a battery radio.[13] Around the St. Boniface Sanitorium, praying nuns filled sandbags next to soldiers trying not to curse as they lugged them. There was a freezing, driving, constant rain. Flood lore has it that one soldier, working 24 hours straight, threatened to plug the Most Reverend George Cabana, then co-adjutor archbishop of St. Boniface Diocese, into the dyke if Cabana couldn't learn to shovel four scoops to the bag.

When people fight a disaster for days, the philosophy "If you don't laugh, you'll cry" can only hold so long. Humans can make a superhuman effort, but only for so long. Frank Rasky, author of *Great Canadian Disasters*, described the night of May 5:

> Rain, sleet and snow, lashed by a fifty-mile-an-hour gale, stung the placid river into a fury. White-tipped waves gouged deep bites out of eight dikes, and the sandbag bastions crumpled and spread like chocolate cake batter in a pan. Four of the city's eleven bridges snapped like clay pipes, and houses were washed out as though a child were wiping a pictured village off a blackboard.[14]

William Hurst, then city engineer for Winnipeg, recalled being summoned to an emergency meeting shortly after midnight. As he and the others sat in the premier's office, the sirens on top of the *Winnipeg Free Press* building began to wail. It was a signal that some of the dykes had failed.[15] Although it wasn't known yet to those at the meeting, one man was dead, drowned in his home when the waves pushed in his barricaded back door.[16]

Hurst later wrote, "The City had exhausted its resources and no attempt could be made to repair the broken dykes but the fight to maintain those left and to retain the utilities and communications was pursued with all despatch." It was decided at the meeting that, henceforth, Brigadier Ronald E.A. Morton was in charge. He had close to five thousand army, navy and air-force personnel at his command. He also had two critical emergencies on his hands. One was the fight to save the power stations and city warehouses of food and supplies. The other was the coordination of relief for people forced from their homes (with the likelihood of more evacuations within hours or days).

This was the situation in Winnipeg when Mrs. Goosen arrived at the Winnipeg General, her labour finally under way. She'd already been through a lot. It was probably just as well she didn't know the entire Maternity Department was about to suddenly change location.

It's not clear from Elinor's various accounts if the army did in fact tell the hospital superintendent it was requisitioning the Maternity Pavilion for flood refugees — and the hospital's move to fill the Pavilion with patients was done in defiance of this — or if army officials simply said something like, "If you're not going to use that empty building, we will." There was a sense, from those who remembered the move, that hospital officials didn't want soldiers and refugees in the new Pavilion because of the ever-present fear of infection; the only way to keep them out was for the hospital to occupy the Pavilion itself.

It is clear that emergency shelters were desperately needed. The *Winnipeg Free Press* reported that close to four thousand flood victims in Winnipeg had fled their homes, and it estimated the rural total was 4,500.[17] It's also clear that decisions about the Pavilion were made very quickly; less than 12 hours after the army had been placed in charge of the city, the move from the General to the Pavilion was under way. Here is part of the account Elinor wrote in her official history of the department:

> Dr. Coppinger [the superintendent] alerted Dr. McGuinness who sent out a call to all members of his professional and nursing staff and to anyone else who wanted to help. The message was that the patients would be moved through the tunnel to the new building commencing at 2:00 p.m. on May 6th. The response was of course dramatic and the move began on schedule. The first patient to leave was a woman advanced in labour.[18]

Mrs. Goosen remembers that ride. Her baby was about to be born and her labour pains were severe. She didn't know where her husband and two small children were or what had happened to their home and livestock. Telephone use was restricted to emergencies, so her husband didn't know how she was either. In the last days of pregnancy, heavy and awkward, she had had to climb in and out of boats to get to the Morris Hospital and then from the Morris Hospital to the train. Now she was being rushed through a long tunnel, about to be delivered by a doctor she didn't know. Although this was her third baby, she was afraid. The nurse seemed upset with her for not answering questions, and the orderly wanted to know if she was excited about her baby being the first one born in the new Pavilion!

But it all ended well. Mrs. Goosen had a healthy baby daughter, born, according to Elinor's history, "in one of the delivery rooms, all proper and correct."[19] Proper, correct, and two minutes after reaching the delivery room. Flood damage was such that it was a month before Mrs. Goosen could return to her home in Rosenort, but she got out of the hospital in four days by promising to take it easy and stay with relatives.

Elinor might have felt a pang of envy — toward Mrs. Goosen or anyone else who could just walk out of the Pavilion and not have to think about it anymore. Elinor's Pavilion problems were just beginning.

It would be impossible to guess, from the short article Elinor submitted to the *Winnipeg Free Press* in 1952, that transferring a maternity department on just about the worst day of the flood was anything but all in a day's work. She wrote that after Mrs. Goosen started off the procession, "patients [holding their charts], supplies and equipment moved in a steady stream through the tunnel, propelled by nurses, orderlies and doctors. By 5:30 p.m., the operation was completed and the patients had been served their supper trays from the kitchen in the Pavilion." She went on to say that the nursing staff "overcame in an admirable way the unfinished details of the new building and it is unlikely that the patients realized how precipitate and unanticipated had been the change of quarters of that Saturday afternoon."[20]

This was Elinor's public persona and voice — proper, straightforward and a touch lofty. Her private thoughts about the emergency, and she had plenty, most of them highly critical, she shared with Gertrude:

> May 6th/50 — We're in a State of Emergency & boy! are my feet tired!! You see, the river was at the '48 flood level by yesterday A.M. & then it started to rain again & *poured* until early this A.M. The dykes that protected all the danger spots were made mostly of dirt, o.a.o. [on account of] our Premier being independent of outside aid, like sandbags, et al & by 5 A.M. today all the dykes had bust: Wildwood in Ft. Garry — 300 homes; . . . Kingston Cres, Victoria Cres. . . .
>
> Yes dear — you guessed it: it took a flood to get us into the new Pavilion! S.B.H. [Saint Boniface Hospital] discharged over 200 patients; their kitchens are all but flooded. . . .
>
> Fortunately the tunnel to it [Pavilion] is the only one that is not flooded. All hands were on deck & I went up about 2 P.M. to see if I could help. In the old dept. there seemed to be more hands than organization, so I got me a load to transport & struggled over to the new Bldg & up to the Case Rooms where they were having 2 cases in a set-up that looked like the back of a junk shop — you know, stretchers & cartons & supplies all over the corridor. I cleaned up a case room, fitted up another, made a bed in a labor ward (maybe not per clinic exactly) & then cached supplies out of sight in cupboards just so the place would look like a hospital again. . . .
>
> There were some funny things happening.[21]

Elinor found watching two of her colleagues struggling to fix the stuck "cheap" delivery tables pretty funny. She thought the practical thing to do would be to get down underneath one and study its mechanics. So she did. Then she gave the table a heave straight out of her shotputting past, and fixed it.

Everyone thought it was amusing when two interns appeared wearing the new hospital "greens." There had been complaints about the old white outfits being far too large. But now "the pants were absolutely skin tight & no hope of them ever sitting down in them — even the flys were gaping between the buttons. We laughed so hard one of the lads began to dribble, which on the light green material did not help our merriment a bit."[22]

On one occasion, Elinor tried to *make* things funny. She marched up to one of the absolutely harassed nursing supervisors and said, "Nurse — I am going direct to Miss Pullen with a complaint: there were *no* coathangers in the doctor's washroom."[23] The look on people's faces — until they realized that Elinor was kidding—caused another round of giddy laughter.

Then there was the matter of the garbage chutes in the new and unfamiliar building being hard to distinguish from the linen chutes. That, added to a new policy of wrapping placentas, meant a few bundles of dirty linen ended up in the incinerator while the placentas went to the laundry.

Charles Templeton, in a televised interview years later, enjoyed asking Elinor about the flood days. He may have considered dribbling interns and laundered placentas inappropriate subjects for Canadian television in 1957. But he couldn't resist asking if it were true that the Winnipeg General incubator plugs turned out not to fit the Pavilion wall sockets. Elinor managed a smile in reply and a crisp, "Well that was quite a trouble."[24] It was the kind of trouble that can only be funny a long time after the fact.

Some of the labour-floor nurses recalled making "preemie jackets" of gauze layers with cotton batting in between. They dressed the tiny babies in these and put hot water bottles in the incubators. When the incubators were deemed warm enough, the plugs were pulled and the delicate cargo sent on its way. Elinor described this to Gertrude:

> After rushing the wee prematures in their incubators through the tunnel into the new nursery the incubators couldn't be plugged in — wrong kind of wall plug. Things like this were discovered all over & the plumber & electrician that had been up all night coping with the flooded basement of W.G.H. were dead beat with the urgent demands on them.[25]

There were urgent demands on everyone, and everyone was dead beat. And the crisis was days from being over. Elinor wrote Gertrude about Jews and Gentiles fighting to save a synagogue, and she described what they were fighting as "an inexorable sheet of dirty water that with supreme calm & indifference keeps spreading out & rising 1 inch per hour, & the crest still away South at Grand Forks [North Dakota]."[26] Elinor was so tired, she wrote, that she could "scarcely move — you know that tearful feeling."[27]

Her tiredness made her more susceptible than ever to worry about Gertrude. Elinor's flood updates are interspersed with remarks like, "I waken in the night & can't get back to sleep. I finish up with you & Murray dead. . . ." A few days later she wrote, "I shall be worrying about the pair of you every mile of the way & every day until I get to see you. I'm still waking in a cold sweat about youse. However, all I can do is commend your safety to God with profound feeling & sincerity. . . . I *love* you." In the letters, Elinor counted down the days until she could see for herself how Gertrude was.[28] In the meantime, she had a big job to do.

Elinor was not head of the department, and the Pavilion was not really hers to command. But as far as she was concerned, McGuinness, who was head, was more interested in saving his house than showing up to take charge. Some of Elinor's colleagues, thinking back, were uncomfortable with this harsh assessment. They described McGuinness as not in good health at the time of the flood, in fact, "pretty shaky."

That may have been true, but where did it leave the Pavilion staff? The following is Elinor's interpretation of events, as told to Gertrude:

Mon. [May 8/50] — You have probably just heard tonight's CBC news so you know our water is now coming down as well as up — both with maddening persistency. . . .

I sought out Miss Johnstone for facts: SBH nurses were sleeping off effects of their evacuation, would later report for duty; some beds still vacant, including privates; 4 labour rooms still vacant. So I sez, O.K. — turn no patients away, put 2 beds in privates & 2 beds in labour rooms if necessary; if no extra beds tell Copp[inger] those were her orders & it was up to him to get the military to requisition beds from Eaton's etc; not to discharge any patient peremptorily if her home was flooded — as many of them are. . . .

The General proper had up in a bad night: SBH patients had arrived sans names, charts, diagnoses, etc., some of them in poor shape, too. No one knew if they were heartcases, post-ops., or recently delivered women. Pretty poor, when they had known evacuation was imminent for 48 hr. . . .

My own opinion about the Lyndale Drive dyke is that it won't stand up now, . . . & when it busts all that gerry-built subdivision will be flattened out like match wood. . . . Love, they are all young veterans who have paid far too much for their new modern homes & it just breaks your heart to contemplate their plight, along with all those who are already sunk. . . .

Jack Lederman told me today the Dean was trying to get in touch with the Pres. — marooned at the U. — to call off our exams this week until the Fall & free 300 young men for flood work. They might as well.

Dear, please send your letters to the office in case I have to move. . . . The puddle . . . is just a few feet short of Balmoral now & we look to be cut off good & proper. I'll go up & live in the women doctor's room at the Pav.[29]

Tues. May 9th/50 — The ground covered with snow after heavy rain all day. No heat & no refrig. o.a.o. the engine of it is running the pump in the basement. . . . The Assiniboine [River] is doing a flank attack on us through the garden & racing with the street end to see which body can flow through the basement windows first — but not yet. . . . The blizzard late this afternoon seemed to want to tidy the city up a bit by covering it with white — stupid idea.

But if you ast me, we're going in circles now! Cause every business & residential block as well as private houses & stores are pumping large streams of water from backed up sewers out into the streets & into the sewers again. No future in it.

I am glad to report that about 50% of the nursing staff of the Heirport [Elinor's nickname for Pavilion] looked this morning as if they had had a bit of sleep last night. Gosh, those girls are tired! They don't know where things are & they are trying to tell strange nurses . . . mostly their problems are small, essential bits of equipment that can't be got & are not easily devised temporarily.[30]

Wed. [May 10/50] — We bin running 'round acting like we were important tonight, o.a.o. I guess we donned a temporary mantle of authority, o.a.o. Freddie 'phoned at 5 P.M. to say he had got all his furniture out & somebody to watch his pumps so he was off to his cottage at the Beach & did I get the MRCOG data O.K. — "Oh, & by the way, you'd better keep an eye on the new Bldg. Good-bye." Not a word about the 4th & 3rd yr exams! However, yon casual remark was good enough for us. After a typhoid shot & dinner, I went up to the Bldg & asked the necessary questions. Discovered, as I suspected, that the woman Resident and the two Juniors had been on call steadily since Sat. & that Otto had been up all night helping them with everybody's cases. . . . So I interviewed Copp[inger] re spelling off our internes with ones less weary before we have a catastrophe. . . . Miss Johnstone came along with her bags, moving into the Bldg to be near if she was needed, so with Copp[inger]'s backing, I ordered her to bed with a sedative; she is so tired she is useless. Saw the Night Supt. who has everything under control for the nonce, & Copp[inger] & I ordered her to deflect all possible cases to Grace Hosp. who have 11 beds, or to the Miseri[cordia Hospital] who have 5. . . .

Four of the 12 examiners didn't turn up this A.M. but we coped with that & slapped the students through in jig-trot time. . . .

Maryland Bridge is now flooded, (The East Kildonan dyke has just bust according to the radio — more evacuations!) which means the Synagogue is surrounded. . . . The water is now over Balmoral St; it is up to the front door of All Saints' Church at Broadway & Osborne. . . .

p.s. The medical students exams are being held at the request of the military because they say they will need those 300 men more next week. The students were grousing this A.M. many of them being water-logged. . . .[31]

ON MAY 10, A DESPERATE CITY ENGINEER TELLS THE CITY'S FLOOD COMMITTEE, "IF WE CAN SAVE THE POWER STATIONS AND THE GAS WORKS, THEN EVERYTHING ELSE CAN GO BY THE BOARD."[32] BRIGADIER MORTON URGES THE EVACUATION OF "NON-COMBATANTS," THAT IS, WOMEN AND CHILDREN. HE WANTS THE POPULATION THINNED OUT AND DEMANDS ON FACILITIES EASED. THERE IS FEAR OF TYPHOID, AND HEALTH-CARE WORKERS ARE ASKED NOT TO WORK ON THE DYKES. A 24-HOUR FREE INNOCULATION SERVICE IS SET UP IN THE WINNIPEG CLINIC.

MORTON PREPARES FOR "OPERATION BLACKBOY"[33] — A PLAN FOR "THE EVACUATION OF 40,000 PERSONS PER DAY BY RAIL, AIR AND ROAD LEAVING 75,000 MEN AND WOMEN IN THE CITY AS A FLOOD FIGHTING FORCE." MORTON'S PLAN INCLUDES STANDBY TRAINS OF FOOD AND CLOTHING, LARGE OVERLAY MAPS OF ZONE HEADQUARTERS, SHELTERS AND EMERGENCY EQUIPMENT.[34] *MACLEAN'S* LATER REPORTS THAT THE PLAN WAS BASED ON ONE DEVELOPED FOR SOUTHERN ENGLAND HAD THE GERMAN ARMIES INVADED IN 1940.[35] THE PLAN WILL GO INTO EFFECT IF THE RIVER REACHES 32.5 FEET ABOVE DATUM. ON MAY 10, THE RIVER IS AT 29.2 FEET AND RISING.

> Fri.[May 12/50] — Aw, Love.... Them urging all women & children that have some place to go to evacuate & me so ready & willing!... I am becoming a bit allergic to the sound of pumps.... How long has this been going on? It seems years....[36]

> Sat.13/50 — I can't phone you tomorrow, Love, o.a.o. they are only taking essential evacuee calls & the circuits are awready jammed. Although we feel it would be an essential call, we might plug a *really* essential one....
> It has been a swell day for our condition — bright sun & a brisk wind from the south. This latter will carry the water & ice further out in Lake Wpg [Winnipeg], but this evening it is over 30 m.p.h. — a bit too much of a batter against the Lyndale dike, I fear. This latter is

now 20 feet high & 40 ft wide at its base. They called for 1,000 volunteers to bolster it last night. . . . As Mrs. Robertson would say, "the water is so insiduous" the way it just keeps creeping up. . . .

People seem to be getting a little sense now & realizing that this is not just a temporary state of affairs that calls for all-out effort 24 hrs per day on the part of everybody, so they are getting some rest & sleep — to the benefit of the total situation. The Emergency Medical Comm. asked me today what job they could put me down for, I said, "Nothing," because I was responsible for the Bldg; they said that was fair enough. My B.P. rises still when I think of [a colleague] phoning me at 6:45 A.M. Wed. to say he had been working on a dyke all night & might be late for the examinations & he felt he should stay with the sandbags. He is a smaller boy kind of man than usual & I knew he was having the time of his life & had probably imbibed plenty liquor during the hours, & would be worse than useless as an examiner. He phoned again at 8 to say he was feeling badly about letting us down & would I "order" him to stay on the dyke. I did so. [He] must be about 54. . . . They are evacuating all possible patients from the General today — to Edmonton. It seems the military are not too sure our power stations are going to remain functioning & they are taking no chances of being caught any shorter than necessary. You know, dear, one just can't believe that all this is actually happening. . . .

Oh, dear! — it has just started to rain![37]

Sunday [May 14/50] — Our situation is "stabilizing" for the nonce, which is a relief. However, we are far from through with the business. You know what happens when the frenzy & excitement dies down — people realize they are tired & lose their enthusiasm for being active & vigilant. . . .

When I was going up in the East side elevator at WGH I was aware of a heavy rushing of water at the bottom of the shaft. "Goodness! Is that water running in or out?" asks I of the operator. "It is running in, Dr.B. — the pumps can't keep up with it." One of our doctors who lives in the 1100 block of McMillan Ave. has been having a bad time keeping his basement dry &, in his district, couldn't understand it & sought the city engineering dept's advice. He was informed that with its loose subsoil, Wpg is literally a floating city now. . . .

There are no lights showing across the river tonight, the residents of those new houses must have lost their fight.[38]

ON MAY 15, OTTAWA ANNOUNCES THAT THE AIR TRANS-
PORT BOARD IS PREPARING AN AIRLIFT CAPABLE OF EVACU-
ATING NINE THOUSAND PEOPLE A DAY FROM WINNIPEG.
THE LYNDALE DYKE DIDN'T HOLD. FEARING MORE DYKES
WILL FAIL, 15 THOUSAND PEOPLE LEAVE THE COMMUNITIES
OF ST. BONIFACE AND NORWOOD.[39]

> Tues. May 16th/50 — Yesterday I . . . was fascinated by a barri-
> cade sign. . . . The water is just a foot short of the top of the under-
> pass, & the sign says: "Closed." A bit tautological if you ast me. . . .
> [Similarly, the *Winnipeg Free Press* carried a front-page warning that
> it was "very dangerous to stand in water and handle live flexible
> electrical cords."]
> The cleaning up of all these dikes off the streets is going to be in
> itself a huge job. . . . Love, it would make you laugh to see Morton's
> reconnaissance helicopter go up from & come down on the Legisla-
> tive grounds without even causing the lift of an eyebrow from
> passersby. . . .
> The river is climbing again tonight & it is raining. However, I
> think we will remain dry here in as much as they have been able to
> keep a fire on since last night — new & better pumping equipment.
> Boy! is it ever nice to have it warm again. . . .
> Last night was another paper marking session. The Medical Col-
> lege was too cold (8 feet of water in the furnace room & below freez-
> ing temps. these nights) so we moved over to the Doctors' Sitting
> Room in the Heirport. Andison, Lyons, Schmidt & Black got off to a
> rollicking start & Best came later in a pontifical mood that we soon
> knocked out of him. I have not laughed so much in months. The
> papers were deplorable — we failed 12 — & as the boners grew &
> were bandied about, our weary spirits got merrier & merrier. All the
> men's wives & families are away & they are lost little boys.[40]

This was Elinor's third swipe in a week at the male
colleagues she normally aligned herself with so closely.
Perhaps the overwhelmingly militaristic and masculine atmosphere surrounding the "Battle of the Red" was getting to
her. The man she really had a problem with was Fred
McGuinness. Elinor told Gertrude, "Love, don't get any

highfalutin ideas about my usefulness around the ossipo et al. All I have done is to make some decisions & accept the responsibility for the policies. They may prove to be all wrong, but at least they remove the stress of the moment & nothing that I have done can be counted as heinous as the behaviour of F.G."[41] Elinor started using military language herself, telling Gertrude she was about ready to sail into battle with McGuinness with "the McIntosh standard flying" — "I am as tall as he is, & have a steadier eye."[42]

At one point Elinor considered moving a couch and six chairs into a room in the Pavilion that McGuinness had reserved for himself. She wanted to create sleeping spaces for the interns, but she thought, "I dassn't get quite that rambunctious."[43] One wonders how much sleep Elinor was getting. Sleeping accommodation for interns was only one of six problems people were waiting to hand over to Elinor that particular day. Elinor wrote Isabel McGill that the Pavilion was confusion worse confounded.

Elinor reckoned that 34 babies were born in the first 64 hours the Pavilion was open, and 73 more by May 16. On the 17, she wrote Gertrude, "No wonder everybody looked a mite jaded. . . . Here it is the end of Wed & this here now river is exactly where it was 5 days ago."[44]

The night of May 18, the river rose to 30.3 feet above datum. Hurst recalled resources being directed to the south side of the city, where McGillivray Boulevard was "holding back what was known as "Lake Morris," a solid sheet of water extending back to Morris, Manitoba." He later wrote, "High winds and rain were threatening to drive this water across McGillivray Boulevard and then overland to the Assiniboine River which would have flooded the River Heights district of Winnipeg."[45]

The next day Elinor wrote, "Rain is promised & is falling & we're not very happy. Aw, Gertrude, we've had enough."[46]

So, finally, had the Red. Massively indifferent to the tremendous damage left in its wake, the water started to recede. The crisis was over and the clean-up began.

It wasn't until this point, May 20, that the prime minister, Louis St. Laurent, visited Winnipeg. Jack Pickersgill, a close advisor to St. Laurent at the time, described the 1950 flood as "an unexpected political problem" for the government. The problem centred around St. Laurent's unemotional statements to the effect that people affected by the disaster could expect appropriate relief from the appropriate channels after appropriate damage assessments were made. This, to those who had been through the physical and emotional upheaval of the flood, did not feel quite satisfactory.[47] In an interview, Jack Pickersgill groaned, remembering. He said that while "Diefenbaker would have *wept, publicly,*"[48] that was not St. Laurent's style. However, the prime minister finally understood that the criticism was hurting the goverment, and he did an extensive tour of the area.

Elinor thought the debate over who would pay restitution was "arrant nonsense" — especially the idea that the United States should pay because that's where the flood started. In the end, the response to the disaster was tremendous. The Manitoba Flood Relief Fund grew to millions of dollars, thousands of claims were settled, and a significant amount of money was left over.[49] In 1988, Pickersgill, still exasperated over the criticism the federal government had taken, said, "We made an enormous deal about it, you know. In the end we had this fund that hasn't been spent *yet!*"[50] The lord mayor of London opened a fund, another was opened in Pakistan. Royal Highland livestock was donated from Scotland and Sheffield sent cutlery.[51]

With the rehabilitation process under way, the return of spring could finally be seen as something other than a wall of water. Elinor wrote Gertrude, "Some baby leaves have come out today & some tulips along the south wall almost & I saw a beautiful oriole."[52]

Elinor's mood was soft. She answered one of Gertrude's letters, "So you were the author of those vague shadow thoughts floating about unnoticed in my mind about playing hookey from the CMA."[53] Elinor was sorely tempted to dodge the annual meeting of the Canadian Medical Association and go straight to Gertrude. Then she thought about the Winnipeg delegates who wouldn't make the annual meeting because of flood losses. Elinor had been through a gruelling time, but compared to them she felt she had got off lightly. The pull to Gertrude was strong, the vacation time well-earned, but Elinor's sense of duty and responsibility was strong too.

This characteristic, and others, including the capacity for crisis management, had not gone unnoted. The decision-making wheels at the University of Manitoba began to turn; the result would break new ground for Canadian women.

Nine

RECOGNITION

▼

We held her in sort of an — awe — you sort of looked up with great respect and awe. She was a little awesome. (Former student)

What a triumph! — oh — what a gal! (Public health nurse)

WHEN ELINOR became the first woman in Canada to head a major medical department some of the letters she received congratulated not only her but also the University. The appointment was described by one woman as a "spectacular performance" on the part of the University.[1] Another correspondent agreed but felt that congratulations to the institution should include "the slightly reproachful question — 'why take so long to decide?'"[2] That it did take an unusually long time is confirmed by another letter describing "the University and the medical profession slowly and painfully sweating it out before they took the plunge."[3]

The plunge — hiring a woman as professor of the Department of Obstetrics and Gynaecology at the University. The

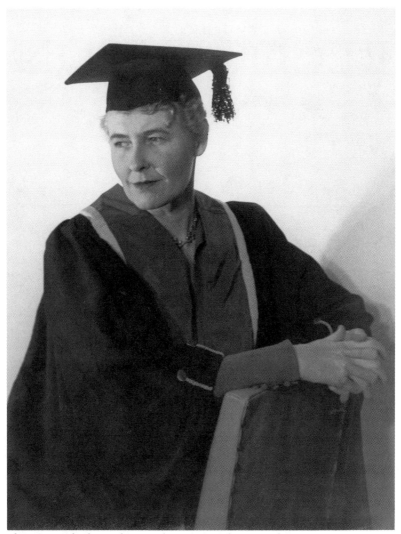

Elinor F.E. Black, professor, obstetrics and gynaecology,
University of Manitoba

appointment was two-fold: whoever was professor would become obstetrician and gynaecologist-in-chief at Winnipeg General Hospital. Why was this decision so difficult? Partly because the Board of Governors had to reconcile the reality of this woman candidate and her credentials with the larger reality of what "women" were perceived to be about.

A Winnipeg columnist who wrote a financial column in the 1950s entitled one piece "A Girl Should Work before Marriage." He advised "young, single girls" to learn an office skill so they would have something to market after their children were "fully grown." (Mothers working before that point, even to "pay bills," were risking "juvenile deliquency and the divorce courts.") The columnist felt that "the women of today tend to stay young looking longer and keep an interest in what is going on," and that was good because "male employers are not blind to that sort of thing." He summed up his advice to girls this way: "If you stay healthy and reasonably attractive, you can put that [office] skill to use later on, and you can help your husband build a nice retirement income. It's a matter of personal choice, of course."[4]

Popular attitudes weren't all that different toward professional career women. Some years after Elinor's appointment, the *Toronto Daily Star* interviewed doctors married to doctors. The newspaper elected to talk only to the women about what this was like. One woman was quoted as saying, "A woman's place, no matter what her profession, is at the breakfast table" and "I have a very understanding husband but I always become Mrs. McEachern after 5 o'clock." Another doctor admitted, "It wasn't always easy for a woman doctor to step out of the hospital and become 'the little woman.'" However, she felt that "she must put her marriage first." And his career, a third woman suggested. She'd put her internship on hold because "naturally it was more important that he qualify first."[5]

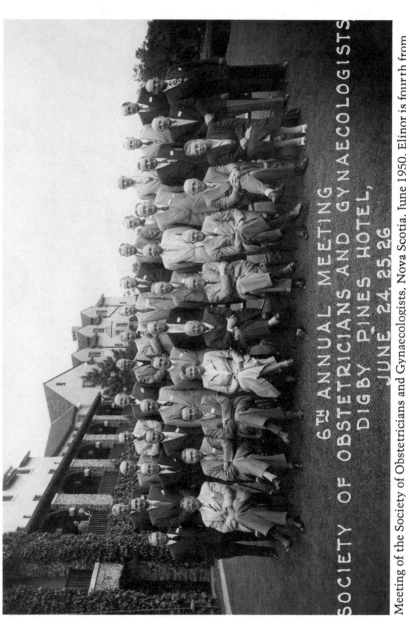

Meeting of the Society of Obstetricians and Gynaecologists, Nova Scotia, June 1950. Elinor is fourth from left, front row.

Most men and women in Canadian society in the 1950s and 1960s shared these attitudes, and the governors of the University of Manitoba were part of society. When they interviewed Elinor, what did they see? The doctor or the woman? Was it a mental struggle to see both at once? Perhaps for some. The woman before them was certainly "young looking," and far more than "reasonably attractive." As those responsible for such an important decision, they couldn't be blind to that sort of thing. What if Elinor up and married? Where would the department be then? Priority number three after her marriage and husband's career? There was a very good male candidate; the race was already a tight one. Why should this board of governors be the one to take the risk? Let some other university make history.

Elinor's friends worried as the process dragged on. One wrote, "I was so frightened that they might overlook you on the grounds of your being a woman."[6] Charlotte wrote Elinor that a family friend "feared that you would not get it on account you are a woman."[7] Elinor must have lost heart at one point. A friend wrote, "I hear that already you are feeling a bit on the shelf, as it were, over the hospital business. Sorry, Old Thing. You've worked so dashed hard through these war years it will be a dirty (stinkin') shame if you are ousted to make way for a mere hombre."[8]

The hombre in question was Dr. Brian Best. His career had closely paralleled Elinor's; the two of them had been promoted to the rank of assistant professor at the same time. Now they were both up for the top job. Dr. Best's advantage, besides the obvious one, was his reputation as a superb surgeon. He was also a few years younger than Elinor, more aggressive, seen by some as more on top of the latest developments, a man with "a brilliant mind."

No wonder Elinor felt discouraged, and, rare for her, actually revealed this to some friends. She was outclassed in surgery, precisely the most macho part of the job. Women were almost completely shut out of surgery as a profession.[9] Dr. Perri Klass, in her book, *Not An Entirely Benign Procedure*, said that the men she did her training with celebrated surgery with back pounding, boasting and "locker-room camaraderie." Klass wrote that they elevated surgery "into the realm of aerospace engineering," and she sensed it was better for her not to "make trouble" by comparing it instead to blanket stitching and quilt patching. (Although having those skills enabled her to pick up certain surgical techniques quickly.) Instead, she "kept [her] mouth shut" and watched the experts "laying complex circuitry."[10]

Elinor did competent surgery (nurses and woman doctors consistently rated her higher than men did) but she had concentrated more on obstetrics. As Dr. Best pointed out in an interview, it's hard to deliver babies day and night — especially night — and specialize in complicated surgery too. "You can't do both," he said. He described gynaecological surgery as his forte.[11]

For Elinor, this situation may have felt a little too much like competing with Donald all over again. In medical school, Donald had won the Chown prize in surgery. Within the family, Elinor had always felt that any competition with Donald was stacked against her, and she made jokes about herself as stupid, the dumb one, the one who never won "real" (academic) prizes. Now she was after the most important prize of her career and competing against her was a brilliant man with a high-status, male-identified ("real") skill that she couldn't quite match.

But Elinor in 1951 was no longer a schoolgirl running after a big brother's approval. Elinor at 46 had her much-publicized Fellowship, her world tour of important gynaecological centres, her publications and her handling of the department during the flood. And, moreso than Brian Best, Elinor had tremendous presence and charisma. This is how people who knew her at that age described her:

> "Majestic-looking."
> "She was stately. Not very many people are stately."
> "Like Michaelangelo's *David*."
> "Like Gainsborough's *Blue Boy*."
> "Like Queen Mary."
> "I stood in awe of Elinor; . . . respect isn't strong enough."
> "You just couldn't not notice her; . . . she had an aura."
> "Commanding."
> "Stunning."
> "We just knew she was such sterling material."
> "Imposing, stately, handsome, . . . a person of such stature."
> "Regal."

Elinor could not help impressing nearly everyone she met, but she would have felt that that was of little value as an end in itself. Elinor's real skill, her own area of brilliance, was handling people. One doctor said, "I don't suppose . . . most people in general *can* be aware of the rivalry and backbiting that goes on [in most hospital departments]. . . . I swore often how lucky I was to be in a department like obs and gyne."[12] Another doctor described working under Elinor's direction as "splendid. Marvelous. Tremendous co-operation. We had the best department in the hospital, I'm sure. People worked together more congenially and more effectively than any other group."[13] These two men felt this happy situation was brought about largely because of Elinor's influence.

An outside opinion, coming from someone who did not work with Elinor but saw her chair a session at an international meeting, echoed the locally held sentiments. The observer found Elinor remarkable enough to mention her in the *British Medical Journal*. He wrote:

> The success of the conference depends more than anything else on the personality and the adroitness of the chairman. Invidious

though it may be to single out one chairman for mention, Dr. Elinor Black (Winnipeg) at the conference on prenatal care, gave a perfect exhibition of the qualities required. She was obviously familiar with the views of her panel, for she was able to draw out contrasting opinions on the same subject. The discussion was kept fluid and any tendency to prolixity was neatly headed off. More humour was injected than is usually shown at scientific meetings, and the audience was kept alert and attentive.[14]

Elinor had the ability to run a smooth meeting and a smooth department. She also had another useful quality. She never blew up at people. Not long before Elinor was appointed chair, an incident took place that she described in a letter to Gertrude. From Elinor's point of view, this is what happened:

Gertrude, I had an *awful* morning today. I was doing one of them new Caesars, my first, on a former Mat. nurse — I told you about how worried I was about her — & Dr. Aikenhead was giving the anaesthetic. I got special orders from him yesterday & wrote 'em down myself so they'd be sure & be right. Ten minutes before the op. I found they hadn't been carried out & I knew he would be madder nor hell 'cause the same thing had happened before. I ran into Miss Johnson & asked her Why??? calmly. She was flying off in a tizzy when a notoriously snippetty staff nurse stopped her about something else & when Miss J. flew at her the nurse cheeked her & Miss J. pinned her ears back & the nurse stamped & burst into tears. Dr. A. arrived on the scene & flew at the scrub nurses, in no uncertain terms. Then he came into where I was scrubbing with blood in his eye. I was being calm & trying to sooth him when in sails Miss J. with her face white with rage & lays into Dr. A. & there were the pair of them shouting at each other. In came Otto who had a peeve on about a case he had last night & he joined in. My taut nerves was so jangled up by this time I wanted to lay down my brush & say "Shut up, all of you! We'll call the whole thing off." — but I knew it would just happen all over again, so instead I asked Dr. A. to please start the anaesthetic, wishing to God I had taken a grain of Amytal 'stead of only 1/2.[15]

This was a minor incident in a day in the life of a hospital. And of course it is Elinor's own version of how she kept her head when all about her etcetera. But it rings true. Not one person interviewed could recall ever seeing Elinor lose her temper at work. She did not yell and she did not leave a trail of tears in her wake. One nurse wanted to point out that Elinor, unlike some other doctors, never threw things at the operating room nurses.

Elinor did get "very — coldly — precise" with people if, as one former student put it, "they failed to meet their obligations." Being reprimanded by Elinor was so intimidating, he said, that anyone who'd experienced it "would have dragged himself [to do what he was supposed to do] if he'd had both legs amputated" rather than go through it again.[16]

Other people tried to explain what it was like watching Elinor use the force of her personality. One woman, a doctor Elinor had encouraged, found herself, totally distraught, sitting in Elinor's office one day. She was there for a pregnancy test; she was still breastfeeding her second child. She said to Elinor, "You know, if I'm pregnant I'm going to go to that fellow on Selkirk Avenue and have an abortion." Looking back at this incident, the woman recalled, "I was partly kidding but I was also desperate." She said Elinor's face "just went like stone." Elinor said only, "We don't do that, you know," but the effect, the younger woman said, "was *chilling.*"[17]

Elinor could, if necessary, cast this chill over an operating room. It was not uncommon for Elinor to be called in to take over a maternity case that was going badly. If the doctor in charge of the case called for help, fine. That was the mark of a good doctor. One doctor said, "We came to know [Elinor] as one to whom we could turn for help when in difficulties, being assured that she would always come at once, be sparing of blame or criticism." That last may have been a mite generous; Elinor was never loathe to offer what she considered constructive criticism.[18]

However, it also happened that Elinor would be called in by someone other than the doctor whose case it was. Let's say a physician with admitting privileges was doing a difficult delivery and a member of the hospital staff got worried about the way the case was being handled. Calling Elinor in meant that the case would be taken out of the doctor's hands. He would have to stand by while Elinor took over.

When Elinor knew she was going into such a situation, she stepped into the case room projecting all the considerable power and authority contained in both her position and her personality. Staff members remembered one instance where the doctor being relieved of a case was full of aggrieved bluster and threats — until Elinor got there — whereupon he instantly became a shadow in the corner of the room.

Not surprisingly, many people, especially students, were in awe of Elinor. But no one recalled being intimidated to the point of feeling afraid of her or trying to avoid her. There was, in fact, some competition to get into her clinics (one-on-one teaching sessions with a patient). Elinor was regularly described as an *"excellent teacher."*

The University governors added up what they knew and what they guessed at and hoped for in terms of potential. They plunged. On November 6, 1951, at a Board of Governor's meeting, the president's recommendation was accepted and Dr. Elinor F.E. Black was appointed professor of obstetrics and gynaecology and chair of the Department of Obstetrics and Gynaecology. The appointments took effect on December 1; the combined salary for the two positions was $4,000 per annum.[19] Definitely a step up from assistant professor — a position that carried an honorarium of $220 a year.[20]

Once again, Elinor's picture appeared in *Saturday Night*

and several newspapers. The appointment was news, a fact that seemed to disconcert some of Elinor's colleagues. One wrote, "The thing that I rather dislike about all the newspaper cuttings and even 'Saturday Night' is the attempt to make of you a trail-blazing feminist and a Famous Woman rather than emphasizing that you are a first-rate obstetrician and gynaecologist and an eminent person quite irrespective of gender."[21] The deputy general secretary of the Canadian Medical Association wrote, "The more militant feminists in the Federation [of Medical Women of Canada] will hail this as a great achievement and so it is. I don't feel that way about it, however, and I prefer to regard it simply as the recognition of a doctor whose contributions to the profession in academic and organizational fields has been outstanding."[22]

Women felt differently. Many who wrote had obviously discovered that roles in society were not assigned irrespective of gender. Elinor's appointment was "hurray for our side!" pure and simple. Two letters even used the phrase "shout it from the housetops." Here is one of them:

Saturday Morn. Nov. 10/51
Dear Prof.
    Last night Isobel Robson whispered the wonderful news to me. I wanted to shout it from the housetops (I refrained — and am still refraining my wild enthusiasm — with great difficulty.) What a triumph! Feminine integrity, ability and intestinal fortitude recognized for the first time in Canada (I would say in North America) that such an appointment has been made — oh — what a gal![23]

One woman felt glad for Elinor and "womankind in general."[24] Dr. Lillias Cringan-MacIntyre, the Calgary school medical inspector who had inspired the young Elinor, declared, "When we say that we are thrilled it is usually an exaggeration, but this time it is definitely an understatement."[25] Another correspondent must have endeared herself to Elinor with this note, "Hurray for our side! . . . I'm sorry it didn't happen before the pavilion went up; then my ride to the OR would have been a mile shorter."[26]

There wasn't much Elinor could do about the design of the Pavilion. And there wasn't a great deal that women, happily claiming her for their side, could do for Elinor. When the newspapers and letters and cards were gathered up, Elinor was in the same position she'd been in for years. It was nice to be named a Winnipeg Woman of the Year, but Elinor's own colleagues were all, or very nearly all, men. Elinor continued her woman/doctor balancing act — doctor side facing out. After 20 years she'd perfected it. It almost never occurred to her colleagues that she wasn't completely one of them.

The extent to which this happpened is shown in some of the letters Elinor kept. One was an invitation to present two scientific papers at a divisional meeting of the Canadian Medical Association. Also, the letter continued, would Elinor "condescend to address the ladies luncheon?"[27] The message seems clear — ladies aren't worth much, and please understand that he wasn't equating Elinor with any such species.

Elinor was known for absolutely deadpan humour, not to mention ironic comebacks. She was liable to react to such a request this way:

> It gives me a glow of pleasure when my male colleagues ask me to respond to this particular toast "The Ladies." I am so used to being included in and absorbed by the generic term "gentlemen" that when my sex is recognized in this public and significant manner, I feel like a dolly who has been cast into a corner for months and then suddenly picked up and brushed up all nice and tidy and sat down at the head of the teaparty table.[28]

Absorbed by the "generic" male is exactly what happened in another instance. A colleague requested that Elinor, in particular, review an article for *Modern Medicine of Canada*. Why her? Because it was magazine policy to solicit comments from "men who are outstanding in the field concerned." The letter indicates he knew who she was; it doesn't indicate he felt any confusion or embarrassment phrasing the request the way he did.[29]

These remarks to Elinor were meant as compliments. But how did she feel when her own dean of Medicine was reported in the newspaper as saying, in 1956, "We can forever dispel the idea that women in medicine are useless?"[30] The dean, Dr. Lennox Bell, had come to this conclusion after recounting a brief history of important women doctors. The spirits of all of them, along with Elinor's, must have sent an ironic bow in his direction.

In 1956, Elinor was running a university department, a hospital department (both without even secretarial help) and delivering close to 300 babies a year. None of this was enough to get her into the Manitoba Club.

A meeting followed by a dinner in honour of the Hon. F.C. Bell, the provincial minister of Health, was arranged by the Manitoba Medical Association (MMA). Naturally it was assumed that Elinor, as head of the Department of Obstetrics and Gynaecology, should and would be there. Just as naturally, this dinner of doctors was booked at the Oak Room at the Manitoba Club, a men's club that women were not allowed to enter.

Elinor wrote in her notes that the organizers "forgot" that she was a woman and this is quite likely true. When they remembered, Elinor must have sensed a high level of discomfort with the idea of changing the club rules. The location could certainly have been changed, but it wasn't Elinor's responsibility to suggest it. She probably would have hated the idea anyway. The location change would create talk, all focussed on her gender, something Elinor worked hard to make colleagues forget about. She bowed out, losing an opportunity to bend the ear of the minister.

The president of the MMA recognized this as "a kindly act" and one that got him off the hook. Embarrassed and grateful, he sent her — roses. And this poem.

> I was sorely dismayed
> When Max said to me,
> "Our staid little maid
> Her face you'll not see."
>
> Then his eyes glared like Hades
> "The rules of your club
> Bar ladies and babies"
> And I felt like a dub.
>
> And more deeply to shame
> Or my grief to compose,
> "This dame's not to blame
> Better send her a rose."
>
> Now no eye will be dry
> When we dine to recoup,
> There'll be a sigh in each rye
> There'll be tears in our soup.
>
> And I fear Mr. Bell
> Will just sob — "nevermore,"
> When we tell what befell
> Our charming Lenore.[31]

If Elinor felt patronized and insulted, she didn't show it. She sent this reply:

> Dear Mr. President,
> No oaken walls surrounded me,
> No party Bell tolled jest,
> No falling of the mercury
> Concerned my poor car's chest—

I sat embowered 'mid roses gay
To sup my slight repast,
Then rapidly was on my way
To reach a meeting, fast.
Said meeting was no tactful ruse
To cover a mistake—
It was a FACT, — and of some use
To give small babes a break.
But, please, DON'T take the roses back
That brought your thoughts to me!
They're beautiful, and salve the lack
Of your good company![32]

Elinor was gracious in her response to the MMA's blunder. With the "dolly at the teaparty" remark, she showed a light touch. There's some evidence, though, that she did not always shrug off the sexism so easily.

In 1952, the *Journal of the American Medical Women's Association* published a one-page profile of Elinor.[33] Elinor cut it out and put it in her scrapbook. There was something else Elinor wanted to keep from that issue, but it was on the same page, other side, as the profile. To have both sides of the page, she needed a second copy of the issue, which she must have obtained. The second clipping is poignant because it is so small, and because of the trouble Elinor took to include it. It reads, "Agnodice, surgeon and obstetrician in Greece and a pupil of Herophilus, is said to have been the first to use the technique of podalic version, on which she wrote a treatise. To avoid notice, Agnodice wore men's clothing."[34]

The "men's clothing" Elinor wore to avoid notice was not literal but psychological and it was as much a part of her professional demeanour as her white coat. When the clothing got too tight, Elinor lashed out.

Generally she did this only in her letters to Gertrude. There was Elinor's swipe at the "smaller boy-type of man" who preferred the masculine atmosphere of fighting the flood to helping with student exams. Elinor liked calling her colleagues "my boys." On one occasion, after a Society of Obstetricians and Gynaecologists of Canada meeting, Elinor wrote Gertrude that a session had been "slick and smart and unnecessarily bawdy." Elinor added in disgust, "Why do they do it?"[35]

Occasionally, Elinor made public statements that indicate she had had enough or perhaps was even trying to get her own back. At a medical meeting in Saskatchewan, Elinor introduced the topic of infertility this way: "The factors underlying infertility are now known to be equally divided between husband and wife, or if one must still provide a sop for the male ego, the best that can be done with the most generous of intentions is to reduce the husband's responsibility to a possible 40%." The tone of the paper suggests Elinor did not appreciate putting women through "tedious and expensive" testing for several months "only to find a state of complete azospermia when the husband finally agrees to be the subject of a most rudimentary test."[36]

Elinor did not even try for generous intentions in a later version of this presentation — a version that included a look at sterilization. Elinor just let fly:

> Supposing the husband is a weak character, shiftless, unable to earn enough to keep his growing family going and, because in the dim recesses of his mind he realizes this, he gets drunk; when he is drunk his wife's nagging doesn't bother him so much and he is full of pride because no matter how much she belabours him he knows that he holds a very triumphal trump card which is his ability to make her pregnant — the only thing in life that he can do successfully. We want to take this one ability of achievement away from him and he resents it.[37]

Elinor must have been thoroughly fed up with the fit of men's clothing the day she wrote that. Although Elinor could be a devastating critic, the sledgehammer was not generally her choice of instrument. Her usual approach was described this way by one of her closest friends: "If I were asked what I would like best of all as a memento of our friend . . . it would be a selection of her letters . . . certain formal submissions which she feels called upon to make from time to time. . . . Closely reasoned and cogently expressed, using when necessary the pondrous phrase, we hear the orotund professorial note. And there is usually included a barb so sharp that even the most pachydermatous recipient must wince."[38]

Just so. This rather orotund tribute described perfectly a response Elinor sent to the editor of *Modern Medicine of Canada*. She wrote:

> The abstract of Alexander Brunschwig's article on radical vaginal hysterectomy for carcinoma of the cervix conveys more enthusiasm for the procedure than does the original article. Brunschwig is a protagonist of the surgical treatment for cervical cancer and his operating experience is very great, therefore it is not surprising that he should extend his technique to include the vaginal approach. However on reading his article one gathers that the leaving behind of involved nodes is not the only "calculated risk" to the operation. . . .
>
> Rather than subject a poor risk patient to radical vaginal hysterectomy for carcinoma of the cervix, it would seem more reasonable to use irradiation therapy. Should the cancer prove to be resistant to irradiation, then surgery would be indicated. The abdominal approach in such a case would still be less hazardous and more satisfactory in the hands of most experienced operators than would the radical vaginal operation in which Brunschwig has gained such facility.[39]

If Elinor considered a practice abuse or bad medicine she often felt called upon to say so. Top of her list seemed to be the rising rate of Caesarian sections and the continuing popularity of hormone treatments.

Elinor's position on Caesarian sections could not have been more conservative. A favourite friend and colleague, in the 1950s and for the rest of her life, was Dr. Alex Andison. He was in perfect accord with Elinor on this issue and spoke about it in an interview:

> A Caesarian section means invading the abdominal cavity, there's always the hazard of infection. There are many complications. It sounds like a straightforward operation and fairly often it is but there are a great number of technical hazards — bleeding, damage to the bladder and other things. It shouldn't — now one child in five is delivered by C-section. . . .
>
> [Elinor] was very concerned. We were both the product of a certain era, . . . the era before antibiotics or sulpha drugs. A patient who had a Caesarian section was at risk of death from sepsis. And we used to see that.[40]

Elinor had indeed seen that. Antibiotics to control infection were available in the 1950s, but Elinor was taking no chances. This irritated some of the younger men, who thought she was stuck in a former era. One doctor recalled that when Elinor was in charge it seemed to him the C-section rate among the public ward patients "was zero." He continued, "And people like me were learning our Caesarian sections purely from the private patients of the other doctors. And every time a staff patient came along, there was some conservative reason why we shouldn't do it. . . . It was very frustrating for a resident to be sort of held back in situations where we thought a Caesarian was needed at the time."[41]

Elinor was aware of the frustration. She wrote, "Our younger colleagues say the years of hardship gave us 'a depression psychology' which made us over-cautious and unprogressive."[42] Her actions indicate that her response to such a charge was, "Too bad." The C-section rate was not just a matter of medicine, it was also, at times, a matter of principle, and Elinor was Frank Black's daughter.

Dr. Andison commented on the former aspect, the medicine. He said, "I think perhaps we had more confidence in our manipulative ability, more confidence in our ability to deliver safely."[43] A younger doctor added this perspective: "Sections aren't that difficult to learn to do competently but forceps are a bit more so. Doctors would get nervous about births not going well, worried about the extent of forceps use and litigation if they bungled it. Also, if they did a section both father and mother had the grateful attitude that [the doctor] did everything he could and saved the baby. If it was a long, exhausting labour that ended in forceps the doctor got little thanks for that."[44]

This was not an unreasonable point of view but Elinor didn't always do what was reasonable. She tried to do — and psychologically muscle others into doing — what she held to be right. She would have seen the argument above as the thin edge of the wedge. She worried as much as anyone else about patients in trouble. She wrote Gertrude, "You know — it's turrible hard, when you & everybody else is awful apprehensive about a patient, not to overtreat them. . . . I have finally adopted a hey-nonny-nonny attitude to try to get everybody to stop worrying — but me. I'm forcing myself into a programme of masterful inactivity."[45]

In Elinor's world, there was no place for C-sections done to earn gratitude. No place either for indulging a private patient who had read about movie stars choosing C-sections and wanted one herself, it sounded more glamorous. Most emphatically upheld of all, though, was the tenet that one did *not* do C-sections because they paid more.

Elinor found no satisfactory explanation for the fact that women who could afford to pay for medical care (private patients) were undergoing proportionally more C-sections than were the ward (or "charity") patients from whom doctors received no fee whether the birth was vaginal or surgical.[46] Elinor was bound to point this out, and did, in a paper on the subject: "A fact which must not be lost sight of is that the incidence [of sections] in private cases has increased out of proportion to that for ward or public cases and is in many instances three times as great. Since the birth rate among private patients is definitely lower than that among public patients, the incidence rate of as high as 9% as given by D'Esppo suggests that indications other than obstetrical are beginning to enter the picture."[47]

A fairly mild comment, for Elinor, but in her department she was in control of this situation, and did not need to bring out the big guns. At least two of the senior members of the department, Alex Andison and Brian Best, felt as she did. As for the younger doctors, they might *think* Elinor was too conservative, but one of them, remembering back, laughed out loud at the thought of any of them telling Elinor so at the time. This doctor remarked drily, "You would be rather reluctant to involve yourself in any criticism."[48]

The question of hormone treatments was different. Those prescriptions, written in doctors' offices in private practices, were between patient and doctor. Elinor felt strongly about this issue, but she couldn't exert direct control over it. Her reaction was to write, to speak out, over and over.

Elinor had two approaches — holistic reasoning and hardline accusation. The first one, holistic reasoning, shows up in almost all her articles, whether she's discussing dysmenorrhoea, endometriosis or the climacteric. Elinor repeatedly suggested explanation and reassurance, and correcting "the over-expenditure of physical and nervous energy" through diet, exercise and proper rest, methods that gave a patient "the satisfaction of being able to cure herself."[49]

This attitude stands in stark contrast to some of the advertising running in the same journals as Elinor's articles. One such ad showed a full-page photograph of a young woman, deeply shadowed, turned away from a baby in a walker who is looking up at the camera in mute appeal. The diagnosis was "delayed postpartum depression," the chief problems described as fatigue and too much to cope with. A series of drug treatments was tried; when the right one was found, the "husband said everything was going very smoothly."[50]

Elinor's dislike of pharmaceutical solutions likely seemed to some colleagues to be all right for women who had painful periods or miserable menopausal symptoms, but a bit simplistic for endometriosis. Endometriosis is a condition where endometrial tissue is found outside its normal location (the lining of the uterus). The tissue can adhere to the Fallopian tubes, the ovaries and other pelvic sites. A review of the medical literature indicates that opinion is as divided today as it was 40 years ago about what causes endometriosis, how to treat it, how pregnancy affects it, and why some women with large endometriotic lesions are free of symptoms and other women have disabling pelvic pain.

Elinor's reaction to the literature was, "The gods must indeed smile at our confused stumbling about in the maze of female endocrinology."[51] She noted that the incidence of endometriosis differed widely in various medical centres and among different social classes. She thought the variance suggested that "one will find what one is looking for." Elinor didn't know, really, what to do about endometriosis, aside from urging a course of treatment "as conservative as is compatible with relief of symptoms." But she knew she didn't know, and she suspected others didn't know either. She thought there was a place for hormones "used with great caution," but she worried.

She worried about "the possible carcinogenic properties of exogenous [not produced within the body] oestrogens administered for long periods" and she worried about combining hormones. She wrote, "The symptoms of endometriosis are relieved by the administration of progestogen-oestrogen substances and palpable endometriotic lesions will regress while the treatment is maintained. However, one must remember that this effect is achieved by completely upsetting the pituitary-ovary-endometrium endocrine complex." What if the assumption — "that the endocrine system is forgiving of all insults" — were false?[52]

Elinor had no "what ifs" about medical management of the climacteric. That, she felt, required no confused stumbling about, and her position on it was straightforward. She addressed one gathering of her colleagues this way:

> Many practitioners prescribe oestrogens routinely when a patient first presents herself with symptoms which might be attributed to the menopause. Unfortunately too often the prescription is given without taking a thorough history and without making a physical and pelvic examination. . . . I deplore the practice of prescribing oestrogens indiscriminately as being contra-physiological, damaging psychologically, and certainly aggravating to possible undiagnosed pelvic pathology. Ovarian activity must come to an end, and the body will adjust to the deprivation. Attempting to forestall or prolong the adjustment is not physiological, and is no kindness to the patient. . . .
>
> Explanation, particularly with recall of the psychological and physiological difficulties the woman underwent at the menarche, will be invaluable in helping her to understand her present discomforts, the causes underlying them, their cyclicity, and their temporariness.
>
> If one can persuade the patient to accept the dictum that each flush means one less to go, her battle is more easily won.[53]

Elinor's own battle — to convert colleagues to her point of view — was not easily won, judging by the amount of effort she put into it. Elinor didn't just address doctors. She took advantage of a request to write an CMA-sponsored article for the *Globe and Mail* to speak directly to the women.

Elinor told readers that it wasn't necessary to "anticipate" menopause; it would arrive at the proper time for each woman. She suggested that women who were having hot flushes should dress coolly, and she added that "highballs and cocktails" increased the intensity of flushes "even though abetting insouciance" about them. Menopausal headaches, Elinor wrote, were warning signals "that the body is not accepting over-expenditure of energy with its previous resilience and suitable slowing down of activities is indicated."

Elinor explained that feelings of depression and irritability were natural because the nervous system was closely linked to the hormone-producing organs. The ovaries were being pushed by the other hormones to produce a period but they no longer could. Elinor went on to say, "As the body in its optimum state acts as a well functioning unit, it is not surprising that when one system of the complex mechanism begins to show signs of diminishing action other systems will feel the effects of that deficiency."

She also explained the rationale behind hormone treatments as one of compensating for the reduction in hormones produced by the ovaries. She said that the treatment "circumvents" symptoms, but it did not help the body. She wrote, "The hormones of the body are interdependent and interrelated and if one is being produced in lesser amounts the others will reduce gradually to maintain a balance and effect a smooth adjustment. The administration of ovarian hormones to the climacteric woman throws out the normal adjustment and prolongs the process unduly."

Elinor ended her article by saying it was the women who feared and tried to fight menopause who suffered, and they need not. She wrote, "The climacteric does not mean that a woman has stopped being useful and attractive. It does not mean sudden wrinkles, grey hair, fat, and the end of sexual activity. It means rather that a woman has set behind her one period of her life and may go on to the next at a slower and more gracious pace, with zest and enthusiasm."[54]

Elinor was wonderfully sane on this issue considering that, during her medically formative years, both menstruation and menopause were listed as "non-venereal diseases."[55]

Elinor preferred persuasion. But she was also capable of flat directives telling others to shape up. In one medical article she said that the "climacteric syndrome" was frequently mishandled, hormone therapy was used too much and too early, and this overuse of such therapy suggested "cupidity."[56] In the same tone, she said that women "making heavy weather" of the stresses of the climacteric would do well to remember what trials they had probably been to their families as young girls entering puberty.[57]

As one of Elinor's former students put it, Elinor "had a real *thing* on hormone therapy."[58] He felt she opposed it too strenuously. Decades later, women's-health activists wrote hundreds of pages documenting and critiquing the *thing* some doctors and pharmaceutical companies had in favour of hormone experiments that turned out tragically for many women: the Pill; diethylstilbestrol (DES) — the "wonder drug" used to prevent miscarriage; depo-provera; hormone replacement therapies to ease the time of menopause, prevent osteoporosis and keep women "feminine forever."[59] Perhaps Elinor dedicated so much energy to this issue because, accustomed though she was to overcoming challenges, she suspected that this was one battle she wasn't going to win.

Elinor did not like being made "sick-at-heart," as she put it, by any kind of bad medical practice. If she was sufficiently offended, she made a foray into an area other than hormone treatments. The more offended she was, the keener the sarcasm, as in this letter sent to the *Manitoba Medical Review*:

Never having been at the Cook County Graduate School of Medicine [in Chicago] I found Dr. R.E. Helgason's account of his recent sojourn there, as reported in the November issue of the Review, very interesting — but also very disturbing. Surely the quoted remark of a staff man at the institution "that the women in labour at Cook County Hospital are in general the most frightened in the world" cannot be true of a centre giving postgraduate training in the gentle art of Obstetrics? Since Grantly Dick-Read had recently been on this continent, one wishes that a marriage of principles and precepts could have been arranged between his extreme views on "natural childbirth" and the apparent assembly-line procedures of the Cook County Hospital as related by Dr. Helgason.

Surely the routine use of pitocin solution intravenously "in normal labors" is an unnecessary and undesirable expediting of labour which is not excusable nor safe even in the fact of an acute shortage of maternity beds? Surely the use of mid-forceps under no other shock-reducing and pain-killing agents than pudendal block and predelivery analgesia is not to be countenanced in these enlightened days of obstetrical anaesthesia? Surely the potentially hazardous procedure of curetting a pregnant uterus deserves more anaesthetic coverage than that obtained by "nembutal, morphine and scopolamine" unless one wishes to return to the inhumane practices of the Russian abortion clinics of twenty-five years ago?

I am sure that Dr. Helgason speaks truly when he says "The knowledge I gained will help me to deal with my obstetrical problems in rural practice," but in the interests of the maternal and infant welfare of our Province, let us hope that he will temper his new knowledge with judgement and mercy.[60]

It's natural that Elinor would link — in opposition — the description of the Cook County Hospital and the name Grantly Dick-Read. Throughout the 1950s, Dr. Dick-Read's opinions on childbirth became the subject of wide media and household debate. The first edition of Dick-Read's book *Natural Childbirth* was published in England in 1933; the book was prefaced with this remark:

But it is generally agreed that one of the most important factors in the production of complicated labor, and therefore of maternal and infant mortality, is the inability of obstetricians to stand by and allow the natural and uninterrupted course of labor. It may be an excess of zeal, or anxiety born of ignorance, but it is an unquestionable fact that interference is still one of the greatest dangers with which both mother and child have to contend.[61]

An expanded edition of Dick-Read's book was published in the United States in 1944 under the title *Childbirth without Fear.*[62] Part of the author's thesis was that much of the pain in delivery was caused by the fear and tension created by modern obstetrical practices such as cold, noisy environments, patients left alone in labour or attended by masked strangers, leg and arm restraints, moving patients from labour rooms to delivery rooms in the last stage of labour and then keeping the woman flat on her back for the delivery. Although Dick-Read repeatedly said that pain-relieving medication should be available to any woman who wanted it, the misconception took hold that Dick-Read had come up with a miracle cure making such medication unnecessary. His book was incorrectly referred to as *Childbirth without Pain* or *Painless Childbirth.* Such a concept was irresistible to the media — and women.

The need for an advocate like Grantly Dick-Read to appear on the scene is evident from Elinor's own letter about the Cook County Hospital and from popular articles such as the one called "Painless Childbirth — Sometimes," published in *Maclean's* in 1950. The article was about a group of women in Toronto who were following — or attempting to follow — Grantly Dick-Read's methods of relaxation and concentration during labour. The article described the reaction of the doctors and nurses as amazed, completely disbelieving or afraid. One doctor, who was delivering a patient for a colleague, was quoted as saying, "I walked in and this woman was lying on the delivery table perfectly relaxed and calm. I figured either she was full of sedatives or had no business being out of the labor room, but when I examined her I discovered she was in the last stage of labor. She argued about it, but we gave her gas and put her down right away."[63]

Elinor would have found this account as disturbing as the one of Cook County Hospital, but on the other hand Grantly Dick-Read was, with one book, turning upside down everything Elinor had learned and practised for two decades. Elinor was stubbornly resistant to changes, particularly sudden or radical ones. She required damned good reasons to change a routine, including proof. As for Dick-Read's speculation that childbirth could be an ecstatic, joyful, spiritual experience, Elinor was unlikely to consider that either interesting or relevant.

Elinor called Dick-Read's views "extreme" in her letter to the *Manitoba Medical Review*. That letter was dated November 9, 1957. The same week, Elinor was interviewed on the fledgling CBC television network, and inevitably the subject of Grantly Dick-Read and "painless childbirth" was on the agenda.[64]

For anyone accustomed to the pace and style of television in the 1990s, the program Elinor appeared on in 1957 comes across as both hilarious and bizarre. There are no voice-overs. The time between shots, and sometimes the delay between what is being said and the relevant shot, gives the impression that one heavy camera is creaking — or being dragged — from right to left and back.

The show opened with dramatic music and a shot of the host smoking a cigarette in a long, black holder. The host introduced himself as Austin Willis, "pinch-hitting for my ailing brother Frank." He went on, "This is 'Close-Up.' Capital *C*. Capital *U*. C.U. That's the spelling — and the approach."

Viewers tuning in on November 3 then saw an interview conducted by Pierre Berton, followed by a studio visit hosted by Joyce Davidson. Elinor's interview, conducted by Charles

Templeton, was the third and last. In a "first for 'Close-Up,'" the story began with a shot of a newborn baby, quickly whisked away. Elinor stepped out of the delivery room, capped and gowned. She shook hands with the interviewer, smiled a dazzling smile and swept her surgical cap back off her head as Templeton asked his first question: "Dr. Black, there are many professions in which I guess it would be a disadvantage to be a woman. I would think in your profession it would be an advantage. Is this true?"

Elinor side-stepped the question completely, answering, "Well, it's a very interesting branch of the profession." Templeton went on to ask about the number of babies Elinor had delivered (over two thousand) and the number the Pavilion handled a year (over four thousand). He asked about the 1950 flood, and if Elinor was married.

Elinor handled the first questions with a kind of open, sunny, crinkly-eyed charm, enjoying especially the drama of telling the flood story. Her chin started coming up when the conversation switched to the latest obstetrical trends.

CT. Do you advocate the [natural childbirth] method?
EB. Well, we go along with the patient if she wants to use the method as far as we think that it is humane and safe. We don't push the method at all here. It's the patient's wishes, if she wishes to use it.
CT. Dr. Grantly Dick-Read, I understand, is an exponent of this method and very strongly believes that most mothers should adopt it. Would you go along with this?
EB. No, we don't go along with Grantly Dick-Read here altogether.
CT. You think this is not appropriate to some individuals because of physiological reasons or —
EB. Yes, well, we appreciate what he has done to remove the fear from childbirth. I think that's very important. But we don't follow his tenets altogether here.
CT. What about hypnotism during childbirth? I've heard this is sometimes used.

EB. Well, I've read about it but we don't practice it here and I can't tell you very much about it.

CT. Do you allow the husband to be present with his wife while she's in labour before she goes into the case room?

EB. Yes, we like to let the husbands in with their wives during labour for a certain length of time but we don't let the husbands go into the case room.

CT. This is sometimes advocated but you would oppose this.

EB. We oppose it here. Very definitely.

Elinor was projecting a good deal of authoritative "Dr. Black" personality by the time she gave this last response. In the next instant, answering a question on how soon women could get up after giving birth, she was all sunshine again. It was very effective.

Elinor did not really give credit where it was due during the exchange on early ambulation. She told Templeton, "We get them [mothers] up early. We find they do much better." It was actually mothers, not Pavilion doctors, who had found this out, mothers like Dorothy Guest.

Mrs. Guest had chosen early June, 1950, as a good time to add a little fresh chaos to the Maternity Pavilion, still coping with the aftermath of the flood. Guest had been reading about "early ambulation" and had told her doctor, "Now *this* is interesting because it's ridiculous; . . . when you get up and go home your legs are like spagetti, you're useless, you need help with the baby. *I'm* gonna try it." The day after Mrs. Guest's baby was born, she got up and had a shower. She said the nurse nearly had a stroke. After an argument with her, and then the head nurse, Mrs. Guest strolled down the hall to explain early ambulation to a friend, who thought it sounded great. The next day, her friend tried it. The friend's doctor was furious.

Mrs. Guest said that doctor tore a strip off her and told her, "You're going to *ruin* your insides, it's going to be a mess," but Mrs. Guest didn't give in. "You just watch," she replied. "I'm going to be fine."[65]

Seven years later, Elinor was agreeing with Guest's assessment on camera. Templeton went on to ask Elinor about learning the sex of the baby ahead of time. Elinor looked thoughtful. She replied, "Yes it's possible. There's been some scientific work done on this whereby some fluid is taken from the uterine cavity during pregnancy and is analysed for cells which show a difference between female cells and male cells. In that way the sex of the baby in the uterus can be determined but it's not a practical method because there's great hazard in taking fluid from the uterus. The woman may go into premature labour and that is not desirable. So it's of scientific interest only but of no practical purpose."

Now Templeton looked thoughtful. "Do you like your work?" he asked. Elinor replied that she did, very much. "Would you advocate this to a young woman who for instance was looking in this direction as a career?" He was getting ready to close his interview and was returning to his opening question. But he didn't know Elinor's history and how little she was prepared to be identified *with* women, much less be an advocate for them, as women. (For them as patients, yes.) She practically shrugged at Templeton's question, and said, "Well if she doesn't mind working hard and losing sleep at nights."

Templeton was well-prepared for this interview, and watching it is like watching two good tennis players. Elinor had the last word, however, and it was a graceful closing. Smiling her winning smile, she told Templeton that even after thousands of births, delivering babies had not become routine to her because, "You are not dealing with cases. You are dealing with a mother and her baby. And therefore there's no routine to it."

Fan mail poured in. "My dear," one letter said. "You really

did miss your calling. You are a *real* T.V. personality." Elinor was told that anyone would be proud to have her as a doctor, that she had the face of an angel, that she must be nice — she could "even twinkle on T.V." Another fan wrote, "I gazed upon you with pleasure and listened to you with delight on the television programme Sunday night. Such a refreshing change from the capering idiots which preceded you. You are a natural for television." One woman couldn't get over Elinor's poise with the surgical cap; "How few stars of stage or screen would dare to remove a close fitting cap during a camera close-up — with no chance to glance at or adjust the hair — but you did it so easily and naturally and of course every hair was in place." Patrick Watson, the producer of "Close-Up," sent Elinor a letter of thanks, calling her contribution to the show "so outstanding." He started the letter, "Dear Dr. Black (or, dear Star, I should say)."[66]

These were the glory years. From 1951 to 1957 Elinor moved in ever-widening circles of admiration, awe and respect. She wore her power and influence easily and used both with integrity. She was in a position to be generous, and she was. The only file almost as large as Elinor's "Letters of Congratulation" was one headed "Letters of Appreciation." Elinor helped a lot of people out, sometimes with an act of compassion, often with money. A patient who had made a tiny installment on a bill had it returned to her marked "paid in full." Some offers to pay were dismissed with a brusque, "I don't charge students." She gave a struggling young doctor her car, saying she needed a new one and he could pay her back whenever he could. She sent a friend who was going through a difficult time on a marvelous trip. Another friend "cried into a towel," overcome by the generosity and speed of Elinor's reponse to a desperate S.O.S.

Elinor gave of herself, not just financially. Many patients wrote notes like, "On those nights when you are hauled out of bed after a particularly tiring day, and on those 'Spring Fever' days, I would like you to remember if possible how very grateful to you we, your patients are." A patient whose baby had died wrote, "I thank you from the bottom of my heart for all that you have done to help ease the blow. No one could have been more wonderful. Thank you especially for showing me my baby girl, as you did. I've relived those seconds a million times since." One woman wrote an exuberant poem, several verses long, the theme of which was, "Long may she live — her sex's pride / To comfort, and with wisdom guide / Her patients, who on every side / Bless Elinor."[67]

For years, Elinor had known only one path — steep and uphill. Now she could enjoy a time of recognition, elegance and plenty. The staff in the Import Room at Eaton's dressed her beautifully (Elinor left it all up to them). She could afford to subscribe to the symphony, which she loved, and to host dinner parties complete with formally uniformed maid. Now the path was smooth and level under her feet, but tragically, a long, dense shadow lay across it.

Gertrude was getting worse, and Elinor's holiday time with her was fraught with anxiety. In 1957, Elinor almost lost her. She wrote to a friend:

> It was straight and sudden heart failure that all but finished her off at 4 A.M. July 16th — the thing we have been fearing since 1944. . . . No hospital bed was available & I was glad because I am quite sure she would not have survived the transportation there. It was nip & tuck the first 24 hours but now she is gaining strength daily, although she has ebbs of energy, which are to be expected, but which distress & discourage her.[68]

Elinor described what she had witnessed as "a catastrophe." She posted herself outside Gertrude's bedroom. One night, Elinor heard a thump. Medical training, steel nerves, strength of character — Elinor was unable to draw on any of these to help her go find out what it was. In what may be the only documented case of it, Elinor was paralysed by panic.[69]

It turned out to be nothing. Gertrude, with Elinor by her side until she had to go back to Winnipeg, survived the summer.

This was how Elinor was spending her vacations — vacations from running a university department and a practice and the Maternity Pavilion.

When the Pavilion opened, the hospital superintendent wrote, "For many years to come it will be possible to accept all cases applying for admission, and it is hoped that never again will the Hospital find itself unable to admit maternity patients because of lack of accommodation."[70] But the baby boom continued unabated throughout the 1950s. Not even a whole new pavilion could cope. One labour-floor nurse recalled being involved in 13 births in one eight-hour shift. She said, "I was delivering on stretchers because the case rooms were all full and then we were backing up with a mother and baby on a stretcher delivered, and another one to be delivered." Another nurse said such a scene happened "fairly frequently."[71] Once again, doctors got into yelling matches with admitting staff over beds.

In the crush, doctors and nurses danced with frustration in front of the Pavilion's elevators. Only the first floor had an indicator saying where the elevator was. On the other floors, the staff had to guess whether or not to bolt for the stairs. This practical aid was missing; but patients were equipped with ultramodern pillow radios, an intercom system connected to the nurses' station. (Neither the nurses nor the patients liked the idea, and the system was largely ignored.)

Many of the patients flowing through the doors of the Pavilion were Elinor's. In addition to all her other responsibilities, Elinor maintained a large practice; the practice paid the bills. Elinor was once paged at Winnipeg Airport where she'd gone to pick up Charlotte. One of Elinor's patients was close to delivering. Grabbing her sister, Elinor told her they'd come back for the luggage. She raced to the hospital, entering the delivery room at the same time as the baby. Everything had been perfectly under control. She wasn't needed. But it was Elinor the patient had chosen as her doctor and Elinor who would get paid. She felt she had to be there.

With this kind of relationship to so many patients, with no secretary to help her with all her administrative work (Elinor even borrowed an office to sit in), with the Pavilion full to bursting every day, Elinor desperately needed her vacations. And, exhaustion aside, it was with Gertrude that Elinor was normally able to be herself, to drop her "cold unemotional doctor" persona. But now with Gertrude so ill, Elinor was working as a doctor all year round.

Elinor's friends knew it couldn't go on. One wrote, "I am heartsick for you. Each summer something prevents you having the holiday you so sorely need." She wrote again, "I am concerned about what this illness is doing to you emotionally."[72] Another friend sent this: "I am concerned about *you*. You ought to spend the next two weeks at a pleasant restful holiday place far from Barrie, before you return to all that awaits you here."[73]

Elinor never left Gertrude one minute earlier than necessary. But what she went through the summer of Gertrude's collapse must have convinced Elinor that her friends were right. She *had* to get away.

▼ Ten ▼

AROUND THE WORLD – AND BACK

▼

Charlotte is fun; . . . as a substitute for you she's not bad!!
(Elinor to Gertrude)

This sister of mine is a natural-born congenital idiot.
(Elinor to Gertrude)

WHEN the Canadian Home Economics Association chose Charlotte as their delegate to the 1958 meeting of the Country Women of the World and the Country Women chose Tokyo as the place to meet, Charlotte decided it was the right time for a sabbatical leave and a world tour. Did Elinor want to come? To Elinor, struggling through another packed year after another non-vacation, nothing could have sounded better. In the Stoughton memoir, Elinor wrote that she saw taking a year off as a good way to bring about her replacement as head of the department.[1] She had had it.

The last time Elinor and Charlotte had got the travel bug, they crossed the Atlantic to see the celebration of the coronation of Queen Elizabeth II. On that occasion, an English cousin recalled, Elinor had argued stubbornly with the hotel staff over removing the flagpole from her window. Elinor was cold and she insisted on shutting her window completely. The hotel staff wasn't having any. This was a coronation; all flags were staying bloody well put.

Not even Elinor was a match for British patriotism during a coronation. Elinor and Charlotte, though, were perfectly matched. By the time they embarked on their trip, this time crossing the Pacific and seeking warm countries, both of them had been heads of university departments for several years. Both of them saw to it that their departments ran the way they wanted them run. Charlotte was called "the General" by students, Elinor was called "the Paratrooper." The entire trip turned out to be a case of immoveable object and irresistible force.

It started out well enough. Elinor got what she called a last-for-a-year haircut. She admitted that she looked like a coconut, but she didn't care. They were travelling cargo ship and Elinor was *off duty.*

Elinor had found someone she thought was ideal to look after her practice for a year. Dr. Jean McFarlane was another of Elinor's protégés. When Dr. McFarlane obtained her Royal College Membership in 1956, she wrote to Elinor, "I shall always be grateful for the help which you have given me; . . . when you asked me to go into practice with you I said that I felt I had to at least get some qualification in order to be in a position to accept — so that I now accept with pleasure and gratitude."[2]

While Jean McFarlane was in England studying, Elinor had received a message from Sir Charles Read, one of McFarlane's supervisors. Sir Charles told Elinor, "I feel I must write you about your protégée. . . . I am sure you would like to know that this girl is really excellent, and everything you said about her has been more than confirmed."[3] Elinor

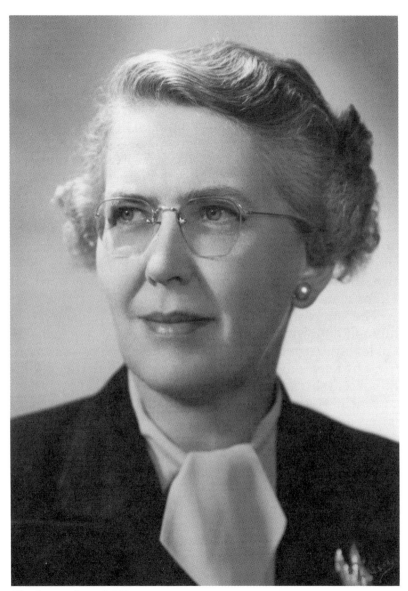

Charlotte, about 1950

had every reason to believe her practice would be in good hands and everything would be fine. The next step was to ask Jack Pickersgill to supply her with a letter of introduction to the heads of Canadian missions abroad. Pickersgill was happy to do this, pointing out in the letter that Elinor was not only a distinguised member of the medical profession but also a close friend, and he would personally appreciate any courtesies extended to her.[4]

So, hair taken care of, practice taken care of, doors abroad primed to open, a cabin full of nine *bon voyage* bouquets, travel literature in hand (including *Five Gentlemen of Japan* and *The Church in Southeast Asia*), they were off.

In Elinor's papers is a small, nondescript cardboard box, originally a little gift box of notepaper. Printed on the front is simply "Around the World, 1958-59." But inside are almost two thousand onion-skin pages — one year's worth of Elinor's letters to Gertrude.

The letters started even before Elinor left Vancouver. On July 24 Elinor wrote, "I've gone away, dear, sure enough — & I'm lonely, but you wait for me & then we'll have some more fun, eh? Keep smiling, please. I love you." A few days later Elinor sent this assurance: "It is kinda hard to leave this here continent you are on, Beloved . . . I shall write you diary letters all along the line."[5]

When the ship pulled out of Vancouver Harbour, Gertrude was not part of the group waving goodbye from the dock. She was in Barrie, thousands of miles away — but something of her was there to Elinor. Elinor wrote, "Sweetheart it is rosemary for remembrance & pansies for thoughts but it's ok — same thing. My 'we's' in letters will have a different connotation now, but you will as always be part of them — just the same as you were the only person I felt on the dock."[6]

Elinor wrote Gertrude almost every day. She told her how, after one "toe-curling" shipboard sermon, she and Charlotte opted for bingo instead. She described her fellow passengers, usually in succinct summations — "a pretty woman who is careful not to disarrange her face when she is talking." Elinor didn't get involved with the other travellers, saying, "I can't ask people too many questions or they will ask me; . . . so far my occupation has remained relatively veiled."[7]

By mid-August, Elinor was reminding Gertrude not to forget the 25th and 26th. These dates in August were highly significant to Elinor. With Gertrude, Elinor used the term "our days" and she wanted Gertrude to remember everything about them. Elinor never explained the reference in her papers, but even after Gertrude died Elinor marked those days in her diary. Gertrude must have felt the same way; one of Elinor's letters reads, "Thank you for your thoughts re our days, M.B. True, *very* true."[8]

The first sign of trouble between Elinor and Charlotte began even before Elinor could decide how she was going to honour these special days. Charlotte had walked with a noticeable limp since she had first relearned to walk. She was unsteady on her feet and often fell, crashing falls that terrified anyone with her. On August 18, Elinor and Charlotte were travelling in Japan, staying at a Baptist House and preparing to walk to a nearby cottage for dinner. Here's what happened:

> I felt for Charlotte's sake that we shouldn't a come. . . . [it was] a good mile of rough road up & downhill, C. with a staff in one hand & me on the other & our hearts in our mouths; the last bit about 1/4 mile was uphill at 60° on a greasy, rooty path. . . .
> [During dinner it poured rain.] In we started [back] with the Chapels along with flashlights. . . . C. fell 3 times in short order hon- est, Love, I was crying inside for her something awful while being stalwart & cheerful outward. Finally she stayed on her knees & slithered backwards down it, me steering her rump around corners. We reached an uphill stretch & proceeded at a snail's pace — but it was sheer nightmare all the way. She fell again.[9]

This incident spelled trouble for the two sisters because Charlotte simply did not acknowledge her disability and didn't allow anyone else to do so. The morning after the disastrous trip home from dinner at the Chapels' cottage, Charlotte got up and rewalked the route by herself.

Elinor was in a difficult position. She understood and admired Charlotte's pride and independence; she had the same traits herself. But what was Elinor supposed to do, let her fall? Elinor wrote Gertrude, "[Charlotte] resents help at times & at other times just expects you to give it automatically — which makes it kinda hard on a feller, see?"[10] Walking arm in arm with Charlotte, Elinor sometimes experienced what she called "the sickening slither" of her sister's arm out of hers as Charlotte's feet slid out from under her. Elinor found herself jumping her arm to her side in her sleep and having nightmares about broken hips. She decided to grip Charlotte's arm in a way that ensured that she could keep Charlotte upright.

Anyone interfering with Charlotte's almost inconceivable pride did not do so lightly. Prior to this trip, Charlotte had once gone on to a meeting after falling and breaking a kneecap. She had chaired the meeting to the end, and admitted to being in any sort of difficulty only when people noticed that she was completely unable to get up and leave. Elinor must have closed her eyes and taken a deep breath before going ahead and overriding Charlotte's wishes on how they would walk.

Elinor's worry and frustration over the situation exploded in a pair of letters to Gertrude. After describing her sister as a "natural-born congenital idiot" in one letter, she went on in the next to say: "Her tumbles are not all on the street, either: she sits on the side of the bed, takes off her shoes & places them in front of her, gets up, trips over the shoes & fair crashes through the floor shaking the whole building. Now wouldn't ya think that having done that once that thereafter one would secrete the shoes under the bed?? Yet I have seen her fall 3 times from this cause."[11]

People who knew only Elinor's "orotund professorial" writing would have been amused by Elinor evoking an image of Charlotte secreting shoes. Elinor in public was so correct — a characteristic that gave Charlotte an opportunity to fight back.

When people asked Charlotte if she'd hurt her leg or had arthritis she answered simply, "Oh no!" That left them wondering and Elinor quite embarrassed. Elinor wrote, "Gertrude dear, it is all very well to say that C. should be taught to accept her limitations — but who's gonna teach her?" Who indeed? Obviously not a baby sister. Charlotte accused Elinor of "destroying her confidence" and taking a patronizing "my good woman" attitude. In the presence of company, Elinor never knew when Charlotte might come out with a conversation-stopper like, "No, I'm not lame, it is just that I fall & that embarrasses Elinor."[12]

This edge to Charlotte was something that could throw Elinor, keep *her* off-balance. And that kept things equal. Once, Elinor was touring Charlotte's new home economics buildings and she picked up a one-handed egg beater. Attempting to work it, Elinor sustained a "foul pinch" on her hand, at which point Charlotte said coolly, "Yes, that's why we have it so our students will know it is not satisfactory."[13] Charlotte was using the same wait-and-sting approach on this trip. Elinor was probably less successful than she thought at being "stalwart and cheerful." Charlotte had known her sister for 53 years and was intuitive about Elinor's feelings. She sensed it when Elinor was "crying inside" for her. Charlotte did not forgive pity.

Elinor longed for Gertrude. She wrote, "Ah Love, I wish we were doing this trip together; we'd be busting with laughter one minute & solemned by superb peace & beauty the next." When Elinor was moved by something, she wrote Gertrude about it, adding, "You & I had a long conversation all day." She also said, "Sweetheart, I have discovered another reason why I am so passionately attached to you & like living with you. It is because you waken me carefully & gently in the A.M. & don't start banging around & opening curtains 20 minutes before I have to get up, see?"[14]

It wasn't all trouble on the trip. Elinor loved Charlotte, describing her as "fun" and "interesting." And Elinor was frequently "solemned," or fascinated or amused by what she saw around her. When the sisters moved on to Australia and New Zealand, Elinor was light-hearted enough to take delight in lambs having breakfast — "their wee tails going like propellors with joy. Quite a few ewes had twins, so they had propellors on both sides."[15]

It was on this leg of the journey that Elinor's track-and-field past caught up with her and caused a bizarre accident. She wrote one of her memoir/stories about it, entitled "The Shark-Fishing Episode off the Great Barrier Reef." The story starts this way:

> One thing we wanted to do particularly was to visit the Great Barrier Reef — such a romantic sounding place which I pictured as being made up of palm fringed turquoise lagoons where girls dancing in reed skirts decorated the edges of the pools. Yes, Cooks could oblige us with a trip up north but we were a bit late to book into one of the regular run small ships that took tourists from the area of Brisbane out to tour the reef islands. However, there was a new ship that had just been completed and had only just begun the regular tour. It was called the Esmeralda and according to its brochure it was a well-appointed converted submarine chaser. It had a crew of six made up of the captain, the engineer, the sailor, the cook and two hostesses; it was not over booked, being newly launched and the whole thing looked like a fine piece of adventure.[16]

Elinor wrote a fuller description of the *Esmeralda* to Gertrude: "She is s'posed to carry 24 passengers, but thank heaven there are only 7 of us aboard. . . . There are 6 comfortable chairs on the small stern deck — not deck chairs — but otherwise one sits on benches. . . . If we want a shower we have to climb on deck, traverse almost the length of the boat & descend another ladder. I have to roll into & out of the upper berth on my tummy & once up there can't lie on my side o.a.o. portholes. . . . We are told that this [boat] has been chartered by a party of 25 Americans — wot a shock they're gonna get eh?"[17]

Elinor summed up the situation this way: "We dunno how that boat gets a Gov't license: no fire extinguishers in evidence; no limitation of passengers carried; no ship-to-shore radio; only the one small dory for the whole ship, & the crew out for a good time."

Part of the good time arranged for everyone was a try at shark-fishing. Elinor was keen; she was good at fishing back home. She described her first attempt:

> For shark fishing, a hook with a two inch shank and a one and a half inch hook tapered to a very sharp fluked barb is used; the line looked like a blind cord with a large chunk of metal which weighed three pounds attached about eight inches from the eye of the hook; sharks swim deep and the heavy weight was necessary to carry the line down to them. The bait was a hunk of old shark meat. This weight made it difficult to toss the hook any appreciable distance from the side of the ship. . . . I hooked a shark and was amazed at the strength of the pull on my line — I struggled valiantly with it but could not play it much as we fished without rod or reels; I was getting it very gratifyingly close to the ship but had not yet seen the thing when my line snapped and I lost my shark.[18]

Elinor contemplated the mechanics of the challenge. She got a new hook and sinker from the captain and thought she would try folding the line and hook across the sinker, holding them in place with her thumb and throwing the unit like a discus well out into the water. Good strategy, poor execution. She threw, her thumb slipped and there was suddenly a large rusty hook with a three-pound iron sinker attached embedded in the muscles of Elinor's upper arm.

Her North Dakota hog-calling yell, "I've caught my-SELF!"[19] brought everyone running. When Elinor was in medical school, she told the yearbook staff that one of her ambitions was to be a ship's surgeon.[20] Now was her chance. Unfortunately, it was her own right arm needing emergency treatment and she was travelling incognito. Even now, she didn't reveal herself as a doctor. Elinor found herself in the ridiculous position of directing the operation based on, she told the crew, what she had learned in St. John's Ambulance classes.

The captain had the presence of mind to realize that they could at least cut the three-pound sinker off, so they did that. Elinor asked Henry, a crew member, to get a pair of pliers with a cutting edge from the engine room. He flew off, "his Dumbo ears giving him speed."[21] Elinor's plan was to get the eye end of the hook cut off, then push and pull the hook through the arm and out.

Elinor needed her right arm in her business and she meant to keep it. When Henry came back with great, big, dirty pliers Elinor didn't flinch. As soon as the eye end was cut, she sent him back for a smaller pair. She wrote, "As Henry pushed on the shank, the flesh over the barb began to tent very encouragingly and I helped it along with gentle external pressure until the barb was through the skin far enough for Henry to pick it up with the small pliers and pull out the hook." Not surprisingly, the captain was moved to remark, "My God! You're good stuff!" to Elinor as she talked Henry through the process.[22]

With the heavy shark hook in pieces at his feet, Henry

decided to carry on in his heady new role. Announcing his own "ambulance-corps" medical knowledge, he began traumatizing the tissue around the punctures in the skin because "this here wound has not bled enough to suit me, we need to get more blood out of the holes." Elinor put a stop to that. When crew members and passengers started pouring drinks in aid of recovering themselves, Elinor went to her cabin to get antibiotic ointment on the punctures as soon as possible. Charlotte followed her there, expressing her sympathy, Elinor wrote wryly, with the comment, "Thank God that happened to you and not to one of the hysterical and neurotic passengers!!"[23]

The next day the ship anchored off an island and Elinor spent two hours "gamboling" in warm salt water. It was the best treatment her wound could have had. Two weeks later, there was some inflammation around the puncture holes, and Elinor's arm gave up a substantial crumb of shark meat — a piece of the bait that had been on the hook. She had no more trouble.

Trouble was brewing, however, between Elinor and Jean McFarlane. McFarlane was turning out to be quite independent, and even, as Elinor continued sending written advice and directives, a little terse. McFarlane couldn't understand why Elinor couldn't relax and have a proper holiday (neither could some of Elinor's other friends who wrote her telling her to forget about work) and just leave her to it. Elinor, on the other hand, had spend 28 years nurturing and building a practice that gave her a living. She was protective of it. Plus, she did not see the younger doctor as her partner; she paid her a salary and saw her as an employee. Employees followed directions.

Like daughters obeyed their fathers? In an interview, Dr. McFarlane said that when she first starting working for Elinor she was young, full of vitality, eager for hard work.[24]

The more Elinor took on Frank's old role of long-distance attempts to control and criticize, the more Jean McFarlane started to act like the proud young Elinor. The two women had a problem, one they would have to deal with when Elinor got home.

Home was getting closer. After Australia, Elinor and Charlotte toured parts of Africa and Italy before going to Britain. In Edinburgh, they dropped in to see Isabelle Pagan, the distant cousin who had cast Elinor's chart years before. If Pagan had decided to do an update, she would have seen a few more challenges ahead. But the astrologer was 91 and bedridden; she probably wasn't doing readings any longer.

Elinor already knew the bleakest part of her near future. Her medical training, not astrology, produced the prediction that Elinor wouldn't have Gertrude with her much longer. After the visit to the Pagan sisters, Elinor wrote Gertrude begging her to "*please* take care o.a.o. Elinor was on her way home and wanted to see her awful bad."[25]

As much as such knowledge is ever any help, Elinor had been prepared for Gertrude's death since she read the specialist's report in 1945. Every summer since had been a gift. As 1959 drew to a close, Elinor knew that Gertrude would not see much of the new decade. Elinor was ready to face that sorrow. But nothing could have prepared her for the way the 1960s would turn the rest of her world upside down.

Eleven

A LOSING
BATTLE

▼

Q. *"Doctor Jones, did I see you on Wednesday last on
Notre Dame in your greens?"*

A. *"Oh no, Dr. Black. It was Thursday."*

WHEN ELINOR RETURNED to her practice in Winnipeg, she
had to face two unpleasant realities. In her absence, gynaecology patients had been moved into the Pavilion. Elinor was
furious; she argued and protested, but, as she wrote in her
history of the department, it was a *fait accompli*.[1] Elinor, who
hated changes, had to get used to this one, and to the new
name — the Women's Pavilion. The second problem was that
she and Jean McFarlane could not agree on McFarlane's role.
In an interview, McFarlane stated simply, "We didn't get
along, at the end."[2] They terminated their professional association.

Elinor was devastated. She poured her heart out to
Gertrude in an emotional letter reminiscent of the ragged
note she had written to Uncle Ivor when she and Aunt

Jeannie had parted in anger. Elinor wrote that Jean felt being a paid employee implied "kowtowing" and she wanted to be an equal partner in the practice. Elinor felt there was no equal way to compare her 28 years in practice with McFarlane's two and a half.[3]

Elinor was still hurting from the damage the world tour had done to her relationship with Charlotte. She watched for each letter from her sister, going first to the signature, looking for "Love, Charlotte." It was over three years before she found it. Elinor also watched anxiously for letters from Barrie. The latest news from there was that Murray's health was failing badly. Elinor didn't think Gertrude would survive Murray's death. Now this. Trouble and defiance in her office.

Elinor's professional life had, for some years, been the place she could at least count on stability, and on being in control. She must have had a great deal invested in making her relationship with McFarlane work. When it didn't, Elinor wrote her distress into her diary: "Had another dreadful session with Jean in p.m. She thinks I'm 100% evil."[4] Elinor was not accustomed to self-doubt or to questioning her own interpretation of events and motives. But so much private and professional turmoil made Elinor feel confused to the point of vulnerability. She asked for help. She called a psychiatrist.

Perhaps all the psychological advice Elinor needed was contained in a letter from an old friend of hers named Connie. Connie wrote, "In one way I was sorry [about the breakup] tho' as I've heard she's very good. Very like you was at her age. . . . I think you need a more dependent person as an assistant."

Connie continued, adding this perspective: "Must be doubly difficult when it's somebody who is smart and particularly when it must all seem to come so easy for her after all your struggles. [It's] because of your early struggle and your impeccable integrity that she is so well accepted now.

You made a secure place for lady doctors but she cannot have any conception what you went thro' to give her the 'security' she demands."[5]

This latter idea was the point of view Elinor took into the psychiatrist's office. *What was the matter with young people today? What had they done to earn anything? What had happened to standards? Everything was changing — for the worse. Values were being lost.* Dr. John Lindsay, the psychiatrist Elinor saw, recalled that the conversation they had was mostly about standards. He said Elinor's were *so* high, "old-world standards." He also said that Elinor saw "things as things to be mastered and fought and corrected." That's not only not surprising, it's virtually a given, for Elinor or any girl who came out of a "Victorian" household to begin a medical career in 1930.

It doesn't appear that Elinor was interested in exploring the first part of her friend Connie's analysis. Elinor may have been upset, but not so distraught as to risk a psychiatrist who might probe too deeply. Lindsay was the man who described Elinor as looking like Queen Mary. He said in an interview that he considered Elinor a "fascinating, regal person" and he admired her. During Elinor's visit, they talked about standards, he suggested Elinor could either change her reaction to the situation or get out of it, and the session concluded with Lindsay lending Elinor a book of Montaigne's essays.[6]

Elinor seemed to have found the experience positive; at any rate, she tried to proselytize Jean, get her to see a psychiatrist too. Elinor recommended Dr. Gerda Allison. Allison happened to be a close friend of Elinor's. Jean declined. Elinor saw Lindsay a second time, but it fell to lawyers to structure a final end to the upheaval.

According to Elinor's diaries, the separation process began in late August 1959 and lasted until May 1960. Right in the middle of it, in January 1960, Murray died.

Elinor did not go to her mother's funeral nor her father's. When the time came, she did not go to Charlotte's. Or Gertrude's. One relative had the impression that Elinor felt funerals were of little use; when someone was gone, he or she was gone. But Elinor could definitely be of use at Murray's funeral. She dropped everything in Winnipeg and left immediately, to render whatever help she could to Gertrude. Elinor was able to stay only four days. She left Barrie, writing in her diary, "Hated to desert Gertrude" and "Nothing but question marks in the future."[7]

Elinor returned to Barrie in the summer. The diary notations are a circle of sadness: "Gertrude awakened me at 3 a.m. with tachycardia [abnormally rapid heart rate]"; "Gertrude had very bad spell of fibrillation"; "Gertrude back in bed & no visitors"; "Am very sad about Gertrude."[8]

On January 12, 1962, Gertrude wrote to Elinor, starting the letter with, "Yesterday became unexpectedly loaded and I missed my conversation with you, Love." She went on to mention visitors, a graduate of the United Church Training School and her missionary brother. She talked of international affairs, asking, "Are we to be defeated again and again in the development of world order by the dollar interests?" She asked about Elinor's news, "How did you make out as referee on Tues. re the beds released by the Rehabilitation Dept in the WGH? You will tell me that when you are here."

She closed the letter by saying:

> When you are here! Think of it. This is probably my last letter to reach you before you leave for Hamilton. There you will be near, and, soon you will be here. Praise be! But we shan't be able to stretch out the hours together as we would like to do. They are sure to run faster and faster, as they always seem to do.
>
> I have been feeling better since Sun. last and hope to continue so from now on. Enough of that internal (infernal) disorder!
>
> Bless you! I love you — Gertrude."[9]

Gertrude died a few weeks later, on February 27, 1962. In a tiny pocket diary, Elinor wrote a stark memorial: "So ends 39 years of love & friendship."[10]

The next day Elinor wrote, "Bewildered by Gertrude's death" and then she did the only thing she knew of that could be of use. She wrote a letter, dated February 28, to the United Church Training School and donated $15,000 to establish a Gertrude L. Rutherford Scholarship. (To give an equivalent donation in 1992 would cost almost $75,000.) Elinor set up the donation so as to remain anonymous.[11]

The *Globe and Mail* noted the scholarship as a news item and listed some of Gertrude's accomplishments. The *Toronto Star* obituary called Gertrude "a pioneering church-woman" who had helped found the Student Christian Movement, the Canadian Council of Churches and a women's training program for full-time work in the church.[12] A church bulletin carried the headline, "A Tribute to a Great Woman," and said that Gertrude's mind and spirit were large, that Gertrude had been a church "statesman with a magnificent grasp of the world church [who] read widely and thought deeply."[13] The article said Gertrude's gift for friendship was tremendous.

It was to Elinor that women who had loved and admired Gertrude directed their grief and their sympathy. One wrote, "[Gertrude] had the happy faculty of making the other fellow try to reach just a little higher and a little deeper into life." Women wrote Elinor that Gertrude "was a great soul" and "an exceptionally wise woman," a woman of "shining goodness," inspiration and strength. They wrote Elinor to say, "You will feel her loss more than anyone & so I write first to you"; "we remember you. Yours had been a great friendship," and "how much we grieve for you in what must be a terrible loss." A terrible loss, an emptiness, a great blank. Women honoured Elinor's love and grief with all these phrases. They thanked Elinor for being a "tower of strength" to Gertrude and for "assisting the dear Lord [in keeping] her on this earth for all those extra years." One woman wrote, "I know how desolate you must be. . . . I am so thankful you have your work, work, as you say, which she had such a hand in."[14]

But how much longer would Elinor have her work? Her work was changing beyond recognition, a reality Elinor intensely disliked. She was coping for the moment, refusing to concede much ground. Helping her, perhaps, was not only Gertrude's memory but also the last letter from Donna Stoughton — another woman who had definitely had a hand in Elinor's career.

Since Pater's death in 1955, Donna had been living in a seniors' residence. She reported herself happy there, as she did everywhere she found herself. A few days before Donna died, she sent Elinor a letter, addressing the 56-year-old doctor as "Childe dear" and telling Elinor one last time that she was a credit to her profession and her family. Donna went on to say that she had written a play in verse for the residents of the home and had scripted herself to play a toy soldier. Donna wrote, "I have to do a dance . . . and I am being outfitted with white ducks, a red coat, and a tall red hat with high airy trimming. I shall look about 7 feet tall."[15]

Elinor, who was so often irritated by the Stoughtons' whimsical notions, was charmed by this image. Donna, even at her age and with her health problems, would spend her final days on earth dancing in a make-believe costume. She was true to herself to the end, and laughed at the residents who called her a "goose." Elinor called her courageous.

Elinor's own sense of self did not falter. The social storm that was "the sixties" was starting to buffet her from all sides, but Elinor could no more retreat from a battle than Donna could be shamed for dancing. And anyone who challenged Elinor's belief system would not be facing a toy soldier.

One of Elinor's more intriguing diary notations reads: "To lawyers at 2 re university suit with a madman."[16] Obviously the suit did not proceed very far; nearly everyone questioned who was around the department in the 1960s was mystified by the reference. But one doctor said he had a feeling it was connected to an incident involving a man who wanted to be in the delivery room with his wife when she gave birth. The man was denied entry. One recalls Elinor's cool rejoinder to Charles Templeton's question about this idea: "We oppose it here. Very definitely."

Having dispatched the "mad" futurist, if indeed that was who he was, Elinor took on the students. She wrote in her diary, "They looked like a bunch of thugs — gave them a blast."[17] Her diary shows that she continued to "bawl them out" fairly regularly. She threw a student out of her class for wearing sandals and no socks, cutting short his argument on the physiological merits of skin that could breathe. Elinor told him he wouldn't be allowed back in until he came around to her way of thinking on socks. Elinor later called a friend and worried about what she would actually do if the student forced the issue. But he didn't. Elinor hadn't lost her touch. She laughed inwardly when he next showed up for class wearing socks of the brightest possible florescent orange.

Elinor wasn't laughing, however, when she wrote this: "Internes lunch mtg re insubordination. They are an undisciplined bunch."[18] Insubordination didn't begin to describe it. One doctor remembered hearing that students had marched into the dean's office, put their feet up on his desk and presented him with a list of demands.

When Elinor was a medical student, Winnipeg Medical Society meetings opened with a sing-a-long; student nurses met every day for 6:30 a.m. prayers; they addressed each other always as Miss Smith and Miss Jones, and they risked being kicked out of the program if seen off hospital grounds in uniform. Nurses stood up for even student doctors, and all doctors rose to their feet whenever a dean or head of department entered a room. No one dared to speak to those higher on the hierarchy unless spoken to — a resident *might* be allowed to hand a department head his umbrella.

Elinor kept a semblance of this practice going in the Women's Pavilion after other departments had adapted to student passion for egalitarianism. When Elinor entered the Pavilion's doctors' lounge, interns still found themselves somehow pulled to their feet, not by Elinor's old guard of loyal staffmen (and one woman), already standing, but by Elinor's own implacable emanations.

The day was inevitable, however, that it no longer worked. Elinor had spied a intern off grounds in hospital greens and later pounced, calling out in ringing tones, "*Doctor* Jones, did I see you on Wednesday last on Notre Dame in your greens?" The student answered, "Oh *no*, Dr. Black." Meeting Elinor's wilting gaze with a mischievous one, "It was Thursday."[19]

Elinor was shaken. She was not prepared, in only her late fifties, to feel like an amusing anachronism. If this hitherto inconceivable conversation could happen, and it had, what might happen next? Young female anaesthetists might keep showing up in her operating room wearing ankle socks instead of nylons. This was undignified, in Elinor's opinion. And then there was the spacesuit.

This plastic suit, invented with the idea of easing labour pains by reducing the difference in pressure inside and outside the womb, was designed to be inflated after the patient was put inside it. One nurse recalled, "By the time you got the patient into it she was just so *agitated*."[20] The nurses got rid of the spacesuit, as they had the pillow radios, by ignoring it.

It was more difficult to ignore the ultimate 1960s symbol. It was everywhere. As one of the clinic nurses put it, "They [students] would reach over to listen to a heartbeat and all that *hair* . . ."[21] Elinor went to the store and came back with hair ties. Another small fire put out, for now. In her clinics Elinor could control the hair but not the rebellious minds underneath. She could handle or dismiss one determined father, one sockless student, one technological invention to conquer labour. Neither she nor anyone could control what these incidents represented collectively. There would soon be another father, and another, banging on the door of the delivery room. There would be another beard-and-sandals turning up to scrub beside her. There would be management of labour technology beyond imagining.

Elinor had loved teaching but now she felt that the students were not receptive to advice like, "Go home and read about it today and come back and do it again tomorrow. Your hands must become much more sensitive." Elinor was irritated, as were other teachers, by students who "turn[ed] aside any sort of telling with an air of boredom."[22] These students, Elinor felt, did not want to look at anything normal, only the abnormal and the unusual. They did not want to be taught, they "just want[ed] to learn . . . by themselves by using their intelligence." Elinor believed that "students [had] to be given some pegs to hang their knowledge on."[23]

Foundations. Elinor believed in them, taught from them, held to them. But the foundations were crumbling. Elinor remembered how hard doctors had fought in the 1930s for the city relief agreement that would pay them a dollar a visit, how thrilled she had been to work for nothing every afternoon at the hospital because it released her from staring at her empty waiting room. Now she saw interns arguing for the right to free parking at the medical college and "issuing ultimatums about their terms of service."[24] She didn't wish her early hardships on them, but she simply didn't understand their attitudes. It was the old question of resistance: "What do you people want, anyway?"

Others were as baffled as Elinor. One friend wrote to say, "Elinor what has caused this complete change of outlook, this lack of integrity, the thing that was so obvious in our parents, it just bewilders me, and it must be perfectly heartbreaking for you after all you have done to build up, or try to build up the right approach to your profession."[25]

When Elinor sat around her quiet office in the 1930s, sometimes reading to pass the time, she may have felt a twinge of amused recognition at a line penned by one of the authors she read. Margaret Lawrence Greene wrote, "The Scots are native exhorters. . . . They think people should be made to be better."[26] Elinor was trying her best. Losing ground at the Pavilion, she took her position to a larger theatre of operations.

In 1961, Elinor, as the first woman president of the Society of Obstetricians and Gynaecologists of Canada (SOGC), had the opportunity to speak out. What better place to shore up the right approach to her profession than a SOGC presidential address? Elinor's address was entitled "The Obsolescence of Leisure," and began with a series of questions.

> Where are we going — so fast and so far? What is the ultimate end of the pace modern man has set himself? Should we take time to ponder these questions or are we inextricably caught. . . . Labour now has a 40-hour week and aims for one of 30 hours. Does this create a sense of leisure in the worker?

Not at all, Elinor argued. It just gave the worker time to work a second job, to buy cars and motorboats and golf bags too full of specialized clubs to carry on foot. Elinor thought society needed a "leisurely, thoughtful amble along a bosky path" but it wasn't taking one because that "would seem so totally unproductive." She said modern man couldn't bear to be alone with himself.

Elinor dismissed the latest architecture, saying it wouldn't enhance "the self-respect of a comfort station." She couldn't see how prefabrication could "uplift the hearts and souls of men." Next, she examined politicians. She had some pity for them. She felt they wouldn't be so easily made fools of by journalists if the politicians didn't schedule three meetings a day in three different time zones, leaving no time to arrange their thoughts before they opened their mouths.

Just as the audience may have started to wonder, Elinor answered the query, "But what have all these questions and ruminations to do with obstetrics and gynaecology?" It was a passionate answer.

> They delineate the milieu in which we practice and teach, and from which we draw our patients. We too are part of this world which has forgotten the necessity and the benison of leisure. What are we teaching our students and residents? Medicine through the ages has been looked upon as a learned profession; the adjective connotes more than manual dexterity, more than the ability to retain scientific formulae and facts. We can teach our residents to be utilitarian functionaries with a fine financial future, or we can teach them to be humane master craftsmen who cherish the patient and not the surgical procedure.

Elinor concluded her speech with the thought that medical journals were proliferating "unconscionably." She felt that doctors were, or should be, capable of reading something other than scientific articles and talking about something other than medicine. They had to find, to be allowed, the time.[27]

That night Elinor wrote in her pocket diary, "*Standing ovation!!*" She had struck a chord. The *CMAJ* printed her speech, and the *Financial Post* used excerpts, missing the point perhaps by using the headline "Slow Down to Go

Ahead."[28] Twenty-four people wrote to Elinor requesting reprints, some of them sending personal letters.

One doctor wrote:

> I have just read your Presidential Address in the *CMAJ* and I hasten to tell you how much I enjoyed it. It is certainly refreshing to read something like it in a medical journal and highly encouraging to anyone interested in civilization to find one in your position taking such a stand.
>
> I am giving it to one of our brightest residents to read, since I have long felt that these residents — whom we are training to replace us — should be something more than highly knowledgeable medical ignoramuses — if you get what I mean.[29]

Another colleague wrote that he was surprised to find such an article in a medical periodical. He was so concerned, he said, about the lack of peace and privacy that he was quitting the rat race and taking Elinor's article with him "to show the rest of the world that there are a few North Americans who are not happy about the mad rush for material possessions."[30]

Elinor's address was her swan song, a perfect note to leave on, a final professional triumph. Elinor was more than ready to take her own advice and slow down. The problem was, the dean wasn't moving very quickly on her letter of resignation.

Elinor's first letter to Dean Bell was dated September 17, 1960. She wrote that a full-time chair had become essential, she wished her resignation to take effect not later than the end of the 1961-62 session, and she would be pleased to go even sooner — as soon as the position could be filled.

Dean Bell's enthusiasm for the task of finding a successor could be summed up in these words he wrote (more like sighed) to the University's president in May 1961: "The first action, I suppose, should be to request the University to agree."[31] Part of the problem, undoubtedly, was in another part of Elinor's first letter: "The current budget of the Department of Obstetrics and Gynaecology will have to be more than trebled in order to engage a full-time Head and Professor and the secretarial and technician assistance necessary for the adequate fulfilment of the appointment."[32]

In 1961, after 10 years of running the department "part-time," Elinor's salary was $5,400 a year. Dean Bell could talk all he wanted about how he hated to let someone go who was doing a great job — he was likely very sincere — but the point was that Elinor was still having to earn four-fifths of her income from her practice, and she was getting older and more tired every year. One candidate for Elinor's job wrote, "I must insist upon no less than $20,000 per annum . . . with assurance of $25,000 per annum at the end of three years. I believe I made it clear to you that the duties of administration, teaching and research do not leave time for supplementation of salary by private practice."[33] Perfectly true, yet the University administration allowed Elinor to do it for years. The longer it seemed content to leave her to it, against her wishes, the more Elinor's irritation turned to real anger.

Elinor's staff was frustrated too, urging that a search for a successor be undertaken "with urgency and the utmost vigour."[34] They knew that Elinor was unhappy being in a caretaker position. It was time, and past time, to move on. The Department of Paediatrics had got a full-time head in 1949, and surgery had had one since 1947. The continuing part-time status of obstetrics and gynaecology reinforced the belief, held by many of the obstetricians interviewed, that their department was the "Cinderella" of the hospital and their profession the Cinderella of medicine.

This notion was strongly present in a 1961 report to the American Gynecological Society. It was published in book form under the title *The Recruitment of Talent for a Medical*

Specialty. One of Elinor's former students wrote to ask her if she'd read it, calling it a "depressing little book."[35] It certainly is.

The book claimed that all approved medical schools in Canada received a questionnaire and implied the schools were reminded about it until there was a 100-percent response rate. The questionnaires went out in December 1958, when Elinor was surviving a shark-hook attack in Australia, so she may never have seen the question, "What is Needed to Recruit More 'Talent' for Obstetrics and Gynecology at Institution of Respondent?"

The premise of the book was that a disproportionately small number of "talented" men went into obstetrics and gynaecology; only 15.2 percent of those choosing ob-gyne were in the top third of their class, and this was "eloquent testimony to the fact that the plight of this specialty is serious." Talented men avoided ob-gyne because "the problems of reproduction were not accorded much dignity in the hierarchy of disease," ob-gyne departments (especially part-time ones) did not do much research, and the "high survivorship" of ob-gyne patients did not pose sufficient challenge for "the talented and intellectually aggressive person."[36]

One chapter of the book, called "Psychological Characteristics Related to Career Choice in Obstetrics and Gynaecology," dismissed ob-gyne students as "hardly distinguishable from those who plan to enter general practice." The authors went on to insult various other groups as well, saying ob-gyne attracted "the fat boy at the bottom of the class who doesn't like to see women suffer," and remarking in passing that students were also tested for "heterosexuality." According to the study, these pathetic ob-gyne students chose their specialty for "curiously" personal or "even emotional" reasons, and that put them in a category with similarly untalented psychiatry and dermatology students — two other fields where vanquishing the death rate was not the primary challenge.[37]

A voice reminiscent of Elinor's is raised in one part of the book: "Emphatic opinion was expressed by some chairmen that research should not be a part of the [obstetrics-gynaecology] residency training program because patient care and clinical training might suffer."[38] Elinor often made such remarks. She also called her field the "art of obstetrics." Any professional climate that could treat her art as this book had done was not one in which Elinor chose to remain as a main player. In September 1964, four years after she had requested it, the University let her go.

Elinor loved her retirement party, writing in her diary, "Beautiful dinner given for me by my men at the Ft. Garry [Hotel]. Orchids, called for by Mervyn [Roulston — Elinor's successor] in a *limousine*, moving speeches by Brian, Buzz, Alex Andison."[39]

Alex Andison was one of Elinor's favourite people and his speech that night conveyed genuine respect, admiration and deep affection. However, the gender confusion Elinor caused all her life by inhabiting her profession the way she did is also there in Andison's remarks. Andison went on to become associate editor of *CMAJ*, where clarity was his business. The night of Elinor's retirement dinner, though, Andison could not quite sort out his thoughts on Elinor's balancing act.

He described Elinor's many accomplishments and added that Elinor had never sought "any concessions on the grounds of her sex." He hastened to add that he didn't mean to present a picture that was "forbidding," that of a "veritable obstetrical and gynaecological blue-stocking." He posed the question, "Must one expatiate upon these male virtues because she has no feminine characteristics? No, indeed, my friends." This can't help but leave the impression that "these male virtues" were in fact synonymous with Elinor's achievements. Andison then made the startling statement, "But if we are to think of our Lady of Honour as a woman . . ."

It would not have been possible, at Andison's own retirement dinner, or Brian Best's or Dean Bell's, for the speaker to say, "But if we are to think of our guest of honour as a man . . ." That would have created puzzled glances and furrowed brows all around. Andison wanted only to pay tribute to Elinor's ability to be a gracious hostess and do Winnipeg proud as a "regally lovely representative."[40] But his remark pointed out, yet again, that thinking of Elinor as a woman did not come naturally to her male colleagues, not as naturally as thinking of her as a doctor.

Dr. Lillias Cringan-MacIntyre, Elinor's old inspiration, had no such awkwardness. She always thought of Elinor as a woman and furthermore she understood the nature of women's work. Cringan-MacIntyre wrote, "You have done wonderful work Elinor and have paved the way for more challenging opportunities for Canadian Medical women. I can well understand that, as a woman, your responsibilities have been even greater than they were for your predecessor and that if your successor is a man, he will have a less strenuous time than you have had."[41]

There was little doubt that Elinor's successor would be a man. The University of Manitoba did not appoint its second female head of a medical department until 1985 — bringing the total to two in its 107-year history.[42] And Dr. Mervyn Roulston, with a properly staffed office and a real salary, did of course have an easier time. Elinor did not feel bitter about that, at first. She hadn't wanted to be a full-time academic; what she *had* wanted was full-time status for her department and she had achieved that.

Elinor was in no mood, however, for any real or imagined slights. The University did not improve its rating in Elinor's books when it sent her the following letter: "Dear Dr. Black," it began, "I am directed by the Board of Governors of the University of Manitoba to notify you that as of August 31, 1964, your appointment as Professor and Head of the Department of Obstetrics and Gynaecology has been terminated."[43]

Elinor was so hurt by this, calling it a "summary dismissal,"[44] that she wrote one of the most subdued replies in all her files: "Without giving offence, I should like to lodge a mild protest. . . . I am sure that both you and the members of the Board are aware that my letter of resignation, stating the cogent reasons for it, has been in Dean Bell's hands since mid-September 1960. For this reason I think the use of the words "your resignation has been accepted" would have been accurate and would be more felicitous for my record in the University files."[45]

By the time Elinor received an apology and a personal letter of appreciation from the president, Elinor had sent copies of the offending letter to friends and relatives. She so needed confirmation of her hurt feelings that she included stamped and addressed return envelopes, exasperating at least one friend, who wrote back, "I could have managed that much for you." The friend added, "Like your brother, I was disgusted with the first letter sent to you from the University. . . . I do not understand why you are being given only $90.47 per month pension for 5 years. If you had been given one for life, you would not have been re-paid, especially as your University salary was so low."[46]

It was right at this time, as this correspondence was going back and forth, that Elinor decided to burn (or shred) all but one of Gertrude's letters. It is a frustrating mystery why she did it, and why at this time, some two and a half years after

Gertrude's death. Elinor's diary states only, "To Pav[ilion] & then spent rest of day destroying Gertrude's letters — a hard job well done."[47]

If Elinor had wanted to protect her relationship with Gertrude from prying eyes, she would presumably have destroyed her own half of the correspondence as well. She did the opposite. She recovered hundreds of the letters she had sent to Gertrude and kept them in files that Elinor assumed were destined for public archives. Perhaps Gertrude had asked her to destroy the letters, but Elinor couldn't bear to until over two years had passed. It's also quite possible that Elinor's tremendous possessiveness of Gertrude could extend this far — to ensuring that no one else would ever hold these letters.

Or perhaps Elinor had never needed Gertrude so much as when she handed over the power and prestige of her departmental position to a younger doctor. Gertrude and medicine had defined Elinor's life. The first loss had been terrible, and without Gertrude, how was Elinor to cope with this second loss, this second great emptiness? Elinor may have destroyed the letters in a resurgence of grief — and rage at grief's necessity. One letter — kept or escaped — remains in Elinor's files. The words, "When you are here! Think of it. This is probably my last letter . . ." may have been too powerful, or too poignant, to be let go.

After Gertrude's death, Elinor returned to the type of vacation that she and Gertrude and a group of others had shared before Gertrude's illness. Finding a welcome with old SCM friends, Elinor rediscovered the joys of a backwoods cottage holiday. Her diary reveals that Elinor was sad and lonely on August 25, but she was also free to once again exploit her physical vigour, a kind of happiness she had set aside for years. Here is Elinor's idea of a perfect vacation: "Made a ladder for the dock. Having a lovely time. / Sawed up a log & cleared some bush. / Felled a tree, sawed it up & went fishing. / Chopping trees & having fun all week. / Walked back to Little Lake & bust a couple of beaver dams. / Back to Little Lake in A.M. & bust some more dams. / Sawed some wood as a farewell gesture. It has been a swell holiday."[48]

It was a shame that Elinor didn't stick to this winning formula. Instead, she took it into her head, upon retirement from private practice in 1965, that she wanted to do another world tour, this time with Frances Ward, head nurse at the Winnipeg Clinic. How to explain the series of trip disasters that started with Elinor and Aunt Jeannie in Switzerland and continued through the visit to Sweden and the tour with Charlotte? This time was no better. (Jamaica, which Elinor attempted in 1968, was worse.)

Putting the wheels in motion, Elinor wrote to Jack Pickersgill for new letters of introduction, describing her travel companion as "a thoroughly reputable person who has been in charge of nursing personnel at the Winnipeg Clinic for over twenty years."[49] Once again, Pickersgill obliged. One of the letters that went out on Elinor's behalf was sent to Jules Léger, then Canadian ambassador to France. Signed by Paul Martin, the letter said simply that Elinor was a good friend of Pickersgill and that she was a medical doctor "*très en vue.*"[50]

Of course Elinor would not be a prominent doctor on the trip, aside from visiting embassies and the homes of other doctor friends. Most of the time she would be plain Miss Black, outstanding only for her trademark travel haircut.

Elinor's friendship with Frances (Frank) Ward ran aground quickly — faster even than had Elinor's relationship with Charlotte during the 1958 trip. By late 1965 Elinor and Charlotte were friends again, and it was Charlotte who received most of the details about this tour. Charlotte's fierce independence had unnerved Elinor in 1958; it appears Elinor had the opposite problem this time.

According to Elinor's letters to Charlotte, Frank Ward couldn't remember where they had been the day before or where they needed to be the day after. She continually asked Elinor questions like, "How do you lock this door?" and "How do you work this venetian blind?" Her response to any wonder that moved Elinor was either "Ain't that somep'n!" or "Isn't that really *something!*" She was always running out of reading material, so Elinor felt she had to take it upon herself to make sure Frank had enough. Elinor took a lot on, saying that she had to do all the accounting and travel arrangements, as well as not allow Frank to amble aimlessly around stores or waste days staying in hotel rooms reading "lurid paperbacks." Such activity, Elinor wrote Charlotte, filled her with "horror."[51]

When Elinor discovered that Frank wore slippers all day aboard the ship and wiped her brow with pink Kleenex, Elinor considered calling the whole thing off. But, Elinor told Charlotte, she had had that out with herself early in the trip and told herself firmly that she had put her hand to the plough, and there was no looking back. She wrote, "One isn't a good friend of a person for over 30 years, [and] lead them into high adventure, only to say, after 4 days of finding out what they are *really* like, 'You don't suit me — you can go home now.'" A different sort of person would, in fact, say something along those lines rather than spend an entire year driving herself crazy. But Elinor chose to see the trip as another opportunity to "build [her] character by saying nothing."[52]

Elinor did blow up at Frank once about not taking any responsibility for the arrangements, calling her mentally lazy. Frank's response to that was, apparently, "I didn't know anything ever bothered you! I didn't think you had a nerve in your body! I'm glad to know you are human!"[53] Obviously,

Frank was not as entirely without resources as Elinor believed.

Head nurses are not generally known to be without resources, neither are they widely regarded as passive, helpless types. Yet Elinor worried constantly about her "thoroughly reputable" friend, even in London, where presumably a grown woman who spoke the language and was an experienced administrator could manage somehow. Elinor wrote Charlotte that she told Frank, "*I* will not leave *you* [in London] unless I am sure that you are going to be properly looked after. That is final & we need discuss it no further."[54]

Oh well. It was not a total loss. Elinor reported being thrilled to be back in Japan, when they visited there. She was also frequently delighted and moved by the occasions of the fine music and singing that she sought out. At other times, Elinor enjoyed examining and sketching unfamiliar mechanical contraptions. And the trip did produce another story/memoir.

In "The Mouse," Elinor and Frank are staying at the Hermitage, a hotel in New Zealand a few hours from Christchurch. Elinor and Charlotte had stayed there in 1959. Elinor wrote in the story that she was looking forward to showing Frank this beautiful spot because she was always hoping Frank might be struck into wonderment at something. As it turned out, Frank had a great time there.

Elinor was just falling asleep when she felt a mouse run across her face. She didn't like mice; she was afraid of them, and of all animals. Doctors learn to bolt out of sleep already thinking clearly, but it's still amazing that Elinor's reaction to her fear and disgust was this: "The mouse had run across my face from right to left so it seemed sensible to get out of the right side of the bed on the supposition that it was hiding somewhere between the bed and the wall on my left."[55] No wonder Elinor's patients said they were in the most level-headed and competent hands possible.

Elinor pulled the bed out and found the "objectionable wild animal." She called the front desk for assistance but got no answer, so she tried to catch the mouse herself, Frank merrily giving advice. When this proved unsuccessful, Elinor knew there was nothing for it but to put on her "nice tartan dressing gown" and go for help.

She had so much trouble convincing the man on staff that he had to do something — "Honest, Mister, there *is* a mouse" — "Well, it won't hurt you" — that Elinor wondered if the man thought she was trying to proposition him. The six-foot doctor and the huge New Zealander succeeded only in finally chasing the mouse out of Elinor's room and under the door of another room, so Elinor insisted on a trap in case the mouse came back. The *man* didn't come back for 20 minutes. Elinor wrote Charlotte that when he did return he was muttering, "I had to damn well go to Christchurch to find one!!" and "I'm bloody well getting out of this before some more fun starts."[56]

He left a baited trap outside Elinor's door, and Elinor pushed the biggest suitcases against the door so the mouse couldn't come back in under the crack. She was safe. She was also saved from something worse — a lost sense of humour. Elinor knew the joke was on her, and she was able to write wryly, "Frank was still laughing. Something had occurred that had really aroused her interest, but it was not quite what I had in mind as a stimulus."[57]

Back in Winnipeg, trip over, Elinor was rarely at a loss for stimulus. She was interviewed on television again, this time a local CBC program. Elinor gave her views on menopause. The producer was enthusiastic, writing Elinor that the discussion was so good she wanted to show it again on another program. Elinor, however, did not feel like a star this time. She wrote in her diary, "To CBC TV to tape talk. . . . I look awful. Old, fat, whisky voice."[58] This is the first time Elinor's reaction to aging appears in her papers; it was a negative reaction that would deepen.

Elinor's appraisal of herself is not borne out by photographs taken about the same time. In the photographs Elinor is elegant and distinguished — and still capable of flashing a cocky twinkle at the camera.

It's easy enough to believe, however, that Elinor *felt* old. She did that interview in 1967, when the whole country was caught up in celebrating itself as 100 years young. A country with a baby boom's worth of children, teenagers and young adults who were proud of being part of a *young* country. Young meant the future, young meant independence and unlimited potential, young meant strength and energy. A British journalist at Expo picked up on the mood of the country, writing with approval, "Canada has made the scene. It would be missed if it went away."[59]

The scene in 1967 included a swinging justice minister talking about the bedrooms of the nation, a steady stream of backpackers hitching across the country, and sex, drugs and rock and roll. Once again, "old hampering conventions had broken down; . . . the young had come into their kingdom." Only this time Elinor was part of the hampering, not the rebellion. When young people parked cars under Elinor's windows and proceeded to have sex in broad daylight, Elinor called the morality squad.

The Pill was having no small impact on the sexual revolution. Elinor, characteristically, believed that the Pill was potentially dangerous to women's health; uncharacteristically, she passed up an opportunity to say so on a panel. She wrote to the organizer:

> I don't think that I am a good person to talk on the Pill because I honestly do not know where my convictions lie. I can't reconcile the assault on one link of the endocrine chain, with potential but as yet

unknown imbalance in other links, with the immediate convenience of contraception. . . . I have been trying for years to form a firm opinion but have been quite unsuccessful; this is why I rarely prescribed the Pill when I was in practice. . . . Sorry to be sticky about this, Ethel, but I think you should have someone who is dogmatic rather than wishy-washy in order to make the best impact on the audience.[60]

Elinor was seeking other audiences, namely the readerships of *CMAJ* and *The Canadian Nurse*. She was still capable of being positively dogmatic about certain issues.

In 1967, *CMAJ* published a report on the Conference on Medical Manpower. One article carried an argument against family doctors being better trained in the social and psychological sciences — not because that wasn't a good idea, but because there was an acute "manpower" shortage, and to suggest that doctors had time for much beyond diagnosis and treatment was "grossly impractical." Therefore, medical training had to be focussed on what the doctors had time for, not what should happen in an ideal world.[61]

Another article expressed concern that, "as economic barriers are lowered" (with medicare), doctors would be overrun with "shoppers" who wanted second opinions, trivial questions answered, curiosity satisfied or scrapes and mosquito bites looked after. The author described with interest a group practice in California that had "automated" a "multi-phasic" check-up:

> Anthropological measurements, electrocardiographs, phonocardiographs, respiratory function tests, chest radiographs, blood pressures, mammography on females, auditory and visual examinations including retinal photos, reflex responses, and complete laboratory examination are done by nurses and technicians, and recorded and interpreted by a computer where possible. The only physical contact which the physician has with the patient throughout the entire procedure is when the pelvic examination and cervical smear are carried out or a sigmoidoscopy is done. On completion of

the examination there is an interview with the physician, who informs the patient of the findings and of the necessary treatment, if any.

The author thought that, if the technicians were pleasant and called patients by name rather than number, this system could work. It was no longer possible, he felt, for general practitioners to "continue to be all things to all people."[62]

Various other viewpoints were expressed in the report, but it was the above two articles that prompted Elinor to sit down and write a lengthy letter to the editor. Elinor did not want what she considered "the basic and fundamental premise of being an M.D. — the doctor-patient relationship founded on the doctor's knowledge of people" undermined. She began:

> For the past few years I have been concerned over the growing tendency in students to think of patients in terms of suitable laboratory tests rather than fixing their minds on what can be done at the moment to relieve the patient of present and obvious distress. This attitude may be engendered because the medical student seems to be increasingly isolated throughout the college years from the ecology of those who are going to need his or her attentions as a doctor. . . .
>
> The tussle for the student's mind and body between the family physician, the specialist and the research investigator is all too evident in the proceedings of the Conference. In this struggle, I am on the side of the family physician or "primary contact" doctor who has established a good relationship with the patient, the family and their milieu. Can we not go farther than "turning out a basic, undifferentiated physician who requires further graduate training to equip himself for whatever field of medicine he chooses to follow?" (Dr. Perkin, p. 1,571). . . .
>
> Why not take it for granted that on qualifying the doctor would automatically go into family practice for two years at least? . . . Anyone who has had responsibility for recruiting candidates for a three-year residency training program in a specialty is aware of the changes of mind that occur as a student matures and progresses through various clinical departments; he is also aware of the advan-

tages to the resident, the patients and the hospital staff if there is a background of general practice.

The student who is definitely research-minded and has no motivation to deal with patients could be directed into studies leading to a Ph.D. in a basic science; or if the investigative urge came upon the student after the training as a family physician, that important training would be a very useful ladder between research on patients and the ivory tower.

Elinor disliked the sound of the "multi-phasic" check-up. She called it "cybernetic medicine" and wondered what possible satisfaction a doctor could get from it. Elinor believed in a doctor-patient relationship that was governed by a sense of mutual responsibility. She ended her letter with this: "I wonder how many members of curriculum committees and medical education committees have had experience in family practice. *Pace*, my academic colleagues."[63]

Elinor was a stalwart defender of the traditional GP; and an even stronger one of the traditional nurse. Elinor sometimes gave the address at nurses' graduation ceremonies. There are several references in Elinor's papers that indicate she had tremendous respect for nurses. One doctor, remembering her student days, said Elinor made medical students aware of any action of theirs that caused unnecessary work for the nurses. Elinor always laid the blame for nursing shortages on the inadequate salaries and recognition that nurses received.

Elinor felt an almost personal sense of betrayal when nurses began to abandon their white uniforms and caps. In distress, she wrote to the editor of *The Canadian Nurse*.

Dear Madam,

I have been an ardent admirer and staunch champion of the Nursing Profession for some forty years, but now there is a trend that I cannot admire. . . .

Elinor felt that nurses, formerly "transfigured" into "handsome, imposing persons" by donning uniforms, would lose authority and pride without them. Patients would have doubts about hospital cleanliness, teenage girls would not be inspired, capping ceremonies would not be "thrilling" nor graduations "splendid."

Elinor must have been truly upset to write the next line: "It might as well be [all abandoned] if the new graduates see that their teachers, supervisors and administrators have packed away their uniforms in favour of looking like a covey of store clerks." Elinor did not usually mix up her public and private writing styles. *The Canadian Nurse* edited Elinor's letter slightly and printed it. Elinor was affronted by the editing, and fired off a second letter suggesting that the changes were made because Elinor had indeed "touched some sensitive spots."[64]

Elinor also wrote to the executive director of the Canadian Nurse's Association to "make a plea" to restore the uniforms. She received a reply referring to the views of psychologists and psychiatrists who advocated "discarding those trappings and regulations which create barriers to a warm and understanding relationship" with patients.[65]

Elinor was fighting a losing battle with the forces of change. On another front, she sent a thousand-word essay to her successor, Mervyn Roulston, written in letter form and divided into sections with subtitles like Patients, Staff Members, Residents. The letter appears to be full of sound practical observations and advice but Elinor didn't help her case with remarks like, "Now that we have a veritable plethora of Residents — compared to the four that the Department of Obstetrics and Gynaecology used to have to struggle along with ..." With such missives she was asking for the brush-off she eventually received: "Many thanks for your continuing interest in the affairs of the Department."[66]

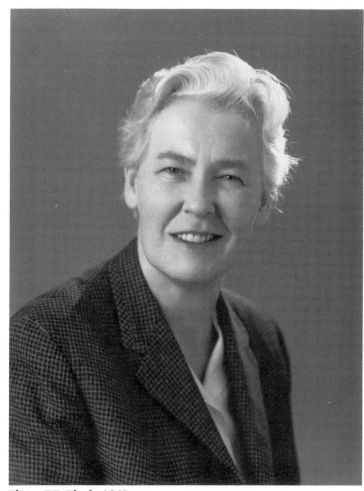

Elinor F.E. Black, 1968

These long letters undoubtedly stemmed from Elinor's belief in acting on principles, speaking out when something is felt to be wrong. There may also have been another reason. Several months prior to this flurry of correspondence, Elinor had been contacted by the Canadian Medical Association. The CMA was preparing a list of nominees for the Order of Canada and wanted her curriculum vitae.[67] Elinor never received this award. Either the CMA decided not to nominate her after all, or her nomination was rejected when the list of recipients was finalized. It must have been a sharp disappointment to a woman who had stacked one achievement upon another since 1936. Could she help but feel that what she had accomplished had been judged and found . . . not that important? These essay-letters have a note of beleaguered defiance: "What I think, what I believe, what I stand for *is* important. I will not *be passed over.*"

Elinor was not swept away by the 1960s. Instead she stood rock-solid in the face of any change she didn't like. It was the only role left to her. The steady stream of students, younger doctors, administrators and nurses-out-of-uniform parted to go around her, joining up again as soon as they were past. Briefly, bumping into Elinor, they at least had to acknowledge she was there.

Elinor's frustration with this role is evident in the pocket diaries. She found 1968 a difficult year. There are two strange notations. Elinor's mother, barely present in Elinor's papers when alive, disappeared completely after her death in 1946. That makes it all the more startling to read, on April 25, "Mother's 105th birthday." A few months later, Elinor decided she would sell her golden-blonde baby hair. She'd kept it for decades; then suddenly sold it for $150. Was Elinor reviewing her past?[68]

Elinor had constant migraines. She recorded the dates of them, sometimes writing "Why?" and "I would like to know what is ailing me please."[69] On her sixty-third birthday Elinor learned she had hypertension. Two days later, her eldest sister, Marjorie, was found unconscious on the floor of her apartment. She died several hours later.

There was not much love lost between Elinor and Marjorie. Marjorie, Charlotte and Elinor were described by one relative as rigid and intimidating in descending order, and that put Marjorie in the category of "absolute tyrant." Elinor had had little to do with Marjorie; there's no evidence she mourned her death. But she did worry a great deal about the effect on Charlotte, who had lived with Marjorie for most of her life. At the time of Marjorie's death, the two sisters were living apart but they kept in touch daily by telephone. Elinor, herself aging and living alone, was chilled by the circumstances of Marjorie's fatal stroke at age 70.

Into this unhappy state of affairs Dr. Dave Stewart's letter arrived like a godsend. Stewart had been one of Elinor's many former-students-turned-friends, a favourite. He had married while still a resident, something almost unheard of in 1942 and not much appreciated by the department head. Elinor had supported Dave's decision and even offered to cover the occasional weekend for him so he and his bride could have some time together. Elinor and Dave shared a sardonic sense of humour and were often of like mind when it came to who and what (including themselves and their own problems) offered opportunities for witty derision. When Elinor had first tried to resign, she arranged for Dave to have first crack at her job.

When Dr. Stewart received the invitation to apply, he was already professor of obstetrics and gynaecology at the University of the West Indies in Jamaica. He chose to stay where he was, and now, a few years later, he no doubt found it amusing to return the favour. How would Elinor like to come down to sunny Jamaica and take over *his* job? Stewart had been offered a three-month assignment in India by the World Health Organization. He was eager to go, but the vice-chancellor of the University was a little fussy about ensuring that someone of similar stature was available to act as a *locum*. Who better, thought Stewart, than a recently retired head but still active member of another Commonwealth obstetrics-gynaecology department?

Elinor was still teaching student clinics two afternoons a week at the Pavilion. She enjoyed it, mostly, and as she told Roulston it gave her something to hang her week around. It was easily got out of, for a better offer, and Dave Stewart's suggestion definitely seemed better.

Fitting neatly into this plan was the fact that the CMA had just begun officially working with the Canadian Executive Service Overseas (CESO) to send doctors to developing countries on short-term projects. CESO president J.-Claude Hébert explained the idea in a letter to *CMAJ* in March 1968, telling doctors that there was no salary, but arrangements were made to pay travelling and living expenses for "the executive and his wife" while they were on assignment.[70] Three doctors, all men, went on projects in October and November. If Elinor went next, in January 1969, she would be the first woman. A minor barrier to break, perhaps, but enough like old times for Elinor to feel back in the swing of things.

Everyone was delighted with the plan. Elinor sounded Charlotte out about going with her and got the answer, "I practically have my bags packed. Certainly I will go to Jamaica."[71] A CMA official wrote Elinor to tell her that the whole arrangement was splendid because it was an academic appointment, one Canadian professor was replacing another and Elinor's sex would appeal to the publicity-minded CESO.

He suggested that Elinor react to any press releases by being "modest, tolerant and cooperative, my girl, and don't give me that Status of Women stuff."[72]

Elinor wouldn't dream of it. She wrote back drily that she would endeavour to exhibit the characteristics required of her. Then she made sure that Charlotte got her plane fare paid for too. Executive and his wife equalled executive and her sister, as far as Elinor was concerned.

Stewart was also writing Elinor enthusiastic letters, "tidings of great joy," in fact. The University, he wrote, was rising to its responsibilities and scraping together an honorarium. He too had some advice to offer: "Now please don't get all altruistic and missionary-minded and protest — it is a very good thing that the University has decided to do this, and the University is very precedent-minded. It is an excellent precedent to be encouraged."[73] Dave also told Elinor that everyone had been warned that she was "*VERY* VIP" and must be encouraged to do what she wanted and not to do what she didn't want. Dave said he would try to sabotage in advance anyone who might not act in accordance with this decree.

Elinor wanted to be briefed on the people she would work with in Jamaica and Dave sent exactly the sort of detailed, breezy and occasionally caustic summation that would appeal to Elinor most. From the midwifery sister ("a remarkable tendency to approach matters on the bias but with extreme accuracy; . . . a tower of strength once you get on her wavelength"), to the bursar of the University ("you will feel the grip of his presence"), to the house officers (interns), Elinor had a cast of characters brought to life for her to mull over before she arrived.[74]

It should have been perfect. Elinor could surely have used a dose of being a VIP again. Moreover, she would get to take Charlotte away from the distress of Marjorie's death, Jamaica would be an adventure and it would be warm, never a negligible consideration in Elinor's books. Sadly, except for a renewed closeness between Elinor and Charlotte, the entire experience went pretty much the way of the trip down — badly.

There was no shortage of bad omens. Elinor left Winnipeg at 9:30 a.m. on December 27, but she and Charlotte didn't arrive in Jamaica until 5:30 p.m. the next day. A blizzard played havoc with plane schedules and prevented the CESO liaison from showing up in Toronto. The same storm — or something — prevented the sisters' luggage from showing up in Jamaica. And Dave Stewart was prevented from showing up at the airport to meet Elinor and help her settle in — he'd been hit out of nowhere by dengue fever. Elinor and Charlotte were met by Ruth, Dave's wife, and Dr. Upendra Nath (Pat) Pathak, senior lecturer in the department.

It might have been partly the dengue, it might have been partly a simple misunderstanding. It could easily have been Elinor's own sense of duty carried to the point of near martydom. Whatever it was, when Dave Stewart left Jamaica for India he left a simple but crucial question not quite clearly enough answered: "Who's in charge here?"

Dave had thought Pathak capable from the beginning of running the department for three months. In his briefing notes, Dave had described Pathak as moving in mysterious ways but almost always coming up trumps in the end. It was more the vice-chancellor who had insisted on someone like Elinor coming in. Dave told Elinor that Pat would have the main adminstration of the department, but he would probably be very glad to have her advice at times, especially as she had no axe to grind. Looking back, Dr. Stewart recalled picturing Elinor as some sort of combination godmother/figurehead about the place who would satisfy appearances and who would, as he had said, be encouraged to do what she wanted — namely teach.

This suited Dr. Pathak. He remembered being given to understand that Elinor was the type who couldn't stand sitting around doing nothing, who liked to work and liked being around young people. Pathak believed he would be acting head, but he would have a senior person to consult with, someone, as he put it, "just coming and going. Not hanging over my shoulder — but there — which I really was pleased about." He thought to himself, "If she wants to keep her hand in she can do a bit of operating. It seemed to me really that all the parties would be very happy."

They might have been. But Elinor appeared to have understood the terms of the *locum tenens* very literally. Dave Stewart was professor and head of the department, Elinor was sitting in for Dave Stewart, therefore Elinor was professor and head of the department in Dave's absence. Technically, of course, she was right. Just right enough to create a problem for Pat Pathak.

He remembered coming in prepared to chair a departmental meeting and finding Elinor in his chair, equally prepared. Pathak felt his performance while Dave was away was crucial to his career. He avoided an open clash but he also said, of his discussions with Elinor, "You see, the juniors used to watch it and I couldn't give way under her onslaught." He admired her though. His first comment, opening the interview, was, "Elinor was a very tough lady, you know."[75]

He admired Elinor's determination to pull her weight, to *fill* what she believed to be her responsibilities as Dave's replacement, her refusal, once she saw the workload, to be a figurehead. Pathak had seen many doctors come to Jamaica, give one lecture at the beginning and one at the end of their month-long stay, and then write the entire month off their income tax as a "teaching visit." Elinor insisted on not getting special treatment, on taking night calls, on doing her share. She wrote her CMA-CESO contact that her activities were more those of an intern than a VIP because it was obvious the department needed the former more than the latter.[76] The problem was, as both the Stewarts and Pathak pointed out, the sheer numbers of cases would have been overwhelming to a doctor many years Elinor's junior.

Pathak said Elinor told him in the beginning that she didn't want to operate much, but she would be happy to teach the registrars (doctors doing a residency). The first week of her stay, Elinor was assisting the registrars in the operating room, and on the second week she arrived in the OR one morning to find the registrar unavoidably away and, Elinor wrote, "nothing for it but to go ahead on me own!!"[77] She hadn't done any surgery for a few years and she was understandably under a great deal of stress re-attempting it in an unfamiliar place where the drugs all had British names and she was having trouble comprehending the Jamaican accent.

Pathak said Elinor "was absolutely shattered at the amount [of cases] we went through. . . . I can remember her coming out absolutely shattered." He quietly arranged to lighten the operating lists Elinor was assisting with, and he put a stop to Elinor being on call at night. She could still be phoned up for advice but she was not to be asked to come in. Pathak said Elinor was not aware of the measures he took.

Elinor and Pat Pathak parted friends. In Jamaica, as elsewhere, Elinor was quick to judge, and critical, and even brittle. But she also displayed the characteristic that had endeared her to others all her life. "She could laugh," Pathak said, remembering. "She could laugh. I can actually see her laughing." When he decided to leave Jamaica for England, Elinor wrote a nice letter of reference on his behalf.

Dave Stewart described Pathak as "a philospher" in his briefing to Elinor, and indeed Pathak had looked at Elinor philosophically. He saw her as tough and aggressive, the type of woman doctor who would say to a patient with bad menstrual cramps, "I don't have that pain. And if I have pain I still work. What are you complaining about?" Pathak felt that he understood why Elinor was like that. He said, "I accepted it as how she succeeded at that time in Canada. You see, I have learned to accept that when, for example, Englishmen went around shooting Indians they were also sending their 12-year-olds up the chimneys in Britain where they suffocated and died. . . . It was a cruel age. People were cruel. They were cruel to women."[78]

Jamaica, for all Elinor loved its scenery ("heavenly"), and many of the people she met there, was a bit cruel to Elinor. The experience pointed out something that Elinor, in her exhaustion, could not deny — she was too old for this game. But what, after 40-odd years of building "as men build" — "With clang and clamor / Traffic of rude voices / Clink of steel on stone / Din of hammer" — what was Elinor, without "the strive to win some outward grace," to do?

Twelve

DAMN THE PASSING YEARS

▼

Grow old along with me! / The best is yet to be.
(Robert Browning)

Browning needed his head read. (Elinor Black)

ELINOR ARRIVED HOME from Jamaica in April 1969 and left again two weeks later for England. Two things contributed to the success of this second trip; she stayed at the Cumberland Hotel "now modernized and *warm*," and, on board the *Empress of England*, she could report "passengers not as crummy as last time." London, Elinor wrote, was "the same old place and I love it." After a few days, she couldn't help but notice that it wasn't *quite* the same. Everywhere she looked there was "the most extraordinary male & female garb on the streets."[1] She had a good time anyway.

Elinor was three days into her return voyage on board the *Empress* when, as she put it, her hypertension "escaped from medication and . . . a transitory ischaemic area occurred in the right cerebral hemisphere; the left leg stopped dragging in about five months."[2] She had had a small stroke. She knew it, as it was happening; with one hand keeping contact with the wall, she made her way slowly back to her cabin, where she could recover alone.

A few months later, Elinor wrote in her diary, "Phoned re X-rays — arthritis and a wedge vertebra."[3] So many people recalled Elinor's swift determined stride; if they were going her direction and wanted to talk they picked up their own pace; if they weren't they got out of her way. She moved like the athlete and deportment-class graduate she was. Now her steps were small, her balance uncertain.

She kept teaching. She and the students seemed to have come to some sort of understanding. She wrote about it to a colleague:

> I must say there are these frequently recurring episodes where I think I have dived neatly into a nice quiet pond only to find myself struggling in the Niagara Rapids, carried over the Falls, and into the maelstrom of present day students knowledge, to surface eventually and swim ashore, dampened and buffetted, but unbowed — and game to try it again.

Elinor asked students "nice straightforward" questions and found herself "inundated with involved answers on electrolytes, enzymology, haematology, and sundry other niceties of pharmacology and biochemistry that had never even been dreamed of when [she] was exposed to those subjects over forty years ago." She wrote, "I stand the onslaught stoically realizing that if the students can explain all this modern knowledge to me, they must indeed know it — or else realize, in making the explanation, that there are a few points they are hazy about. However, I can usually get my own back by asking them a simple question about patient care — which gives me a chance to tell them what one does *for the patient*.[4]

Elinor even saw a funny side to her situation. She said students used so many new and unfamiliar eponymns (conditions with a person's name, such as Parkinson's disease) that "us old folk . . . pass among us the question 'What is that condition?' as if we were playing an old-fashioned parlour game."[5] (The same humour came into play in dimly lit restaurants. If Elinor couldn't read the menu, she just pulled a flashlight out of her purse to help her.)

Elinor's diary still had the occasional "tamed a very smart alec med student to a state of acceptance & appreciation" or "tore strips off all the Residents,"[6] but she was just as likely to report that students were well-groomed, enthusiastic and ready to return to her clinics. There Elinor taught them "only old-fashioned things that . . . computers don't seem to know about."[7] She said that the fact the students came back to her was good for her ego.

Even better for her ego was the news that the University of Winnipeg was going to give her an honorary doctorate. Her diary reports that she was "stunned . . . still excited about Lld" and finally "came all unstuck and blubbed."[8] Charlotte knew what this meant to her sister, and she came through with flying colours by attending the special convocation and also sending this note:

Dear Babe —
 I am so very much pleased by the honour that has come your deserving way. And that it is your confreres who have brought it about. I called Donald right away and told him — did not suggest that he would be present but he did say it was good that one member of the family would be there. He may come around to thinking of going yet. Can you imagine the joy and gladness in the hearts and on the tongues of The Stoughtons and of Daddy's shoulder-straightening pride.
 Well I'm doing it all.[9]

Charlotte had written something similar when Elinor became head of the department — "Daddy would be proud." Elinor's mother's pride was not mentioned on that occasion, or this one. Charlotte, evoking Frank and the Stoughtons, was heading up rather a ghostly delegation, but Margaret would not be present, even there.

It was the last happy time the two sisters had together. The following summer Elinor and Charlotte had "a splendid row." The fight was likely over Charlotte's fragility, which had increased, and her iron determination to keep doing whatever she wanted, which had not decreased at all. Elinor took the opportunity to get "some home truths said," and Charlotte threw her out. The sadness came several days later. Elinor wrote, "She seems to have broken something inside me."[10]

Something was starting to break inside Elinor. Younger women, who had admired and even idolized her, would visit her and come away shocked at the depth of Elinor's bitterness. Not at Charlotte — that was worry stretched to fear — but at her "golden years." With the LL.D. and all her Fellowships, Elinor had 28 letters after her name. She had chosen them, fought for them, using intelligence and will as her weapons. They had brought her public honour and prestige, contact with men and women who were her equals, opportunities to give of her best. The letters hadn't cheated her, they'd done all that letters could do. But Elinor couldn't shake the feeling that *something* had cheated her, that somehow it wasn't fair that her letters should prove such poor company in the end.

All her working life, in an environment that divided men and women and practically forced exceptional women to choose sides, Elinor had needed her technique of being one of the boys. In retirement, she was unable to let go what no longer served her. "I don't get on with women," she still said, to women friends. "I've spent all my life with men." The pattern, so tightly woven over so many years — how to discern the responsibility for the design? How to change it?

"You'll be so lonely," Elinor said to friends about to retire.

Elinor didn't get on, at all, with her arthritic spine. She blamed it on years of difficult deliveries, and she felt tricked by it and by old age in general. "I'm tired of fighting," she snapped. Often in a crotchety mood, Elinor indulged in will revisions, cutting out several relatives and the Winnipeg General Hospital, orginally marked for two-thirds of her estate. Later she put most of the relatives back in but not the hospital. The two-thirds went to the arts, something that had never let her down.

Tired or not, Elinor fought on. She was often in fine fighting trim on the days she wrote her friend Alex Andison, who had left Winnipeg. She sent him the following bulletins:

> Yesterday was the conference at St. B. and it was entitled "Modern Treatment of Stress Incontinence" which, after being dribbled on for some 46 years, I decided I must learn about. . . . Didja know that 50% of the cases of stress incontinence occurs in college girls? . . . Didja know that the uterus should always be removed, whether done from below or above? Boy! you shoulda heard Fothergill hammering on his casket!! Well, there is this to be said about it: it is a good way to get rich — and some of these college girls are going to be in a very bad way. . . . Perineal exercises were just mentioned en passant as there is no money in them, of course. I made some remarks about post-partum exercises but did not trust myself to get started on anything else. I walked out.[11]

> You will know that our doctors have been brought to heel. I am glad, but I wish that it had been by someone other than that fatter, flabbier, more slug-like effigy . . . who services as our Minister of Health. Maybe now some of the padding will be discovered too. All the money I make in the OPD I have in a special account which will provide my bail money when they catch up with me for all the Medicare cards I sign for patients whom I have not examined. When I remonstrated about what I feel is a dishonest practice I was told that

if I didn't sign them another Staff member, who had not even been in the clinic, would sign them, that it is my right to sign them as a University teacher. Curious reasoning — and I am complimented on my "productivity!!!" Maybe some of these rip-offs will come to light now and be remedied. When I have a speculum in a patient, I can see no reason whatever for my being paid an extra fee because I do a Papanicolaou smear; sure the cost of a spatula and a slide is involved, but so what? But I keep quiet because I do not have a wife and family and $90,000 house and mortgage and two cars and two snowmobiles and a cottage at the lake and a sail-boat and a launch. [12]

If Elinor had indeed kept quiet it must have been a rare impulse. She was more likely to pull something like this: "The Caesarian section rate in Manitoba has risen 400% since 1972. These are the figures which Peddle produced from the 'print-outs' from SBH and when I asked what this increase had to do with the Medicare Card, Arthur chastised me privately saying that I shouldn't have asked as there were people from the Commission there and I said I didn't care o.a.o. the figures were too telling."

Elinor wrote that to Alex, and went on, sarcastically:

> Now look here Andison!! What makes you think that your judgement is sufficient for you to deliver that baby properly?? The parents have not had an exhaustive and thorough interview with the geneticists; You have not had ultrasound done to tell you what the gestation is; or where the placenta is; you have not done amniocentesis levels; you have not had daily oestriol levels done; you have not done weekly Oxytocic Challenge Tests; you have not monitored the foetus throughout labour AND you plan to deliver the baby *vaginally*. [13]

Alex Andison, who shared her values, who shared her humour, became Elinor's last confidant/correspondent. It was a type of relationship Elinor knew well. They exchanged news clippings and conference literature, writing sardonic comments in the margins. Alex's wife, Molly, fussed gently about Elinor's health and eating habits, and Elinor teased her with updates on how poor both were.

Elinor's eating habits *were* poor. She had never learned to cook, having waited until 1966 to even try, at which point she said to herself, "Why are you doing this?"[14] Elinor understood one kitchen implement — the pressure cooker. Any dinner that didn't come out of there was liable to be "roast chicken still in the shell" or angel-food cake "o.a.o. protein."

Elinor and Alex commiserated about the current state of obstetrics, about winter, about politics, departmental and otherwise. Andison might open his mailbox to find a blistering 1,500-word account of a meeting Elinor was at, entitled "Miasma Arising from the Lecture at the Last Staff Meeting" and carrying the advisory, "This is not a letter, does not require an answer and does not necessarily need to be read." Another day he would find, "My sympathy goes out a bit to Jimmy Carter these days who has found that nobody else wants to play his game of sweetness and light and live happily evermore if he had used his noggin he woulda known this afore, like" or, "As to Dief using the same hymns as Churchill did, that is *damn cheek*."[15]

Elinor was comforted by the knowledge that Alex at least would be in general agreement that Anne Murray should never have accepted the Order of Canada in a "pantsuit"; that Stan Knowles was the only honest member of Parliament (although even he was slipping by sending out some personal Christmas cards with "the frank on them rather than the Queen"); that *no* MP should yell "Shut up, you!" in the House; that René Lévesque was a very smart cookie indeed and needed watching; that there was more than one *éminence grise* running the postal union and the horn-tangling would result in misery for the letter-sending public; that if God had wanted us to go metric He would have given Jesus ten disciples.

Alex and Elinor commiserated, most of all, about aging. Alex wrote, "I received an invitation just yesterday to attend an organizational meeting for senior citizens, they will pick me up and give me my lunch and all. Oh dear, it comes hard!"[16]

For Elinor, once so vital, it was ill health that came hardest. When she was young and vigorous and striding through her rounds, she used to shake her head at the tenacity of some of the old people who were hospitalized. She told Gertrude once that they could "straight-arm the Angel of death beyond all estimations."[17] In 1975, Elinor went into hospital. She had diagnosed herself as having an aortic aneurysm, and the day after her diagnosis was confirmed she underwent surgery.

An aortic aneurysm is extremely serious. An aneurysm, a sac-like widening in the blood vessel, can rupture or lead to blockage of the vessel. The vessel in this case was the aorta, the main trunk of the arterial system. Elinor's aneurysm was 12 centimetres long.

Perhaps Elinor flexed her shot-putting arm as she was being wheeled into the operating room. The Angel, if it was hovering about, didn't stick around. Not this time. Elinor said later that a nurse told her she came out of the anaesthetic simultaneously moaning and telling herself to "stop it!"

Elinor recovered, refused any attempt to make her a professor emeritus because she wanted to stay on staff as a salaried worker, and went back to teaching clinics. Clinics were easy; she was just doing what she loved. Everything else was getting harder. She wrote Andison:

> Browning needed his head read. The "spin-offs" of age are deplorable. The mind becomes a sieve on top of which everything rests comfortably until one wants something, like a name or an article, and one goes to pick it up and verbalize it when the thing sinks through the mesh, not to surface until some time later. Bones and

joints ache, especially in the mornings; . . . they make swing doors much heavier than they used to and the jars are harder to open and the ground tends to be incontinently irregular sometimes and after years and years of counting the hours until I could get back to my bed and sleep I now find myself wide awake at 5, 5:30 or 6 which seems an awful waste of time.[18]

Elinor had time, as she hadn't had for years, to brood. She finished the Stoughton memoir in 1971, and handed it out to several friends, pressing them into service as "editors." She went over her papers, sometimes writing explanatory or directive remarks on them, sometimes putting in more last names. She thought about what her life had been and what it might have been if the will of her parents and Donald had prevailed so many years ago.

Donald. Close to 50 years after Donald had told her that women were a nuisance around medical schools, Elinor hadn't got over it. Elinor wrote Alex that Donald was jealous of her LL.D. because "he was always opposed to women in medicine, particularly his baby sister and then I made the mistake of making kinda a success of it."[19] She and Alex often exchanged books, or recommended titles, and Elinor wrote, about one, "Well you are welcome to 'Zen and yon motor-cycle.' . . . I tolerated it mostly until the later part when he got into the 4-letter words to make it sell and then I thought: To hell with it! I sent it to Donald for his birthday as a mind-expander, which he badly needs."[20]

Elinor wove similar remarks into the friendly, newsy letters she sent to Harold, Donald's youngest son. The letters show genuine affection for Harold and his family. Elinor sent them large cheques, sometimes to help with dental bills, sometimes for no special reason. Mixed up in the generosity and the interest was criticism like this: "Ever since 1923 I have spent more of my time with men than with women and the only man with whom I cannot carry on a sustained conversation is my brother; I get a topic going nicely and then say: 'What do you think?' and he says yes or no. This is probably my fault because he was very opposed to my going into Medicine ('women were a nuisance around the College') and then life was tactless enough to make me a success — all of which sounds like arrant nonsense, of course, but the subconscious is a strange thing."[21]

It sure is. Did Elinor ever wonder what she was doing, criticizing Donald in letters to his son? Did she ponder the role of the subconscious in her relationship to Donald's daughter Meta? When Meta was thinking of medical school, Elinor promised financial and moral support. But when Meta opted for marriage, a family and nursing instead, Elinor virtually dropped her. Meta did not choose Elinor's path and Donald had tried to block it. Elinor was unforgiving of both, but Donald, from the evidence of the durability of this 50-year-old wound, must have represented something more than himself. He was the first male Elinor struggled past; he came to symbolize every male, and every patriarchal structure Elinor took on thereafter.

Harold Black wrote in a letter that he thought his father, especially in later years, deeply regretted his estrangement from Elinor. He added, "I found some old letters from Dad written during Elinor's last years. Each one reports the latest news of her and expressed considerable concern. . . . I always had the feeling that he was very proud of his little sister's accomplishments. . . . I know Elinor felt very much in his shadow as she went into medicine."[22]

Of the Black family members who offered opinions on the subject, none expressed any doubt that Donald was likely to have been against Elinor becoming a doctor. "However," Harold wrote, "unlike his sisters, Dad could and did change his mind."[23] If Donald did change his mind, Elinor never knew it. One relative sighed, "I think it would have been balm to her soul" if Donald had ever looked at Elinor's contribution and said to her, "I was wrong." But Donald was a product of his time — and of his stiff-necked family upbringing. In thinking over the voluminous correspondence between Elinor and her siblings that is in Elinor's papers, not a single case springs to mind of an apology or admission of wrong-headedness. Pride.

Elinor had one fight left. In 1972, after a particularly bad fall, Charlotte had moved into a seniors' home. She kept up her independent lifestyle and, within the home, organized group discussions based on news stories she culled from various sources. Elinor thought this "social work" was good for Charlotte and good for the others, but it sounds like it occasionally got slightly out of hand. Elinor wrote one relative that Charlotte "had made Mrs. Smyly cry" trying to get her to respond to the assembled newspaper items. Elinor added that Charlotte did not seem "to think it right that they should *not* be interested."[24]

Charlotte's determination to bend whatever circumstances she was presented with to her own will prevailed through a series of strokes. She needed more nursing care, and she needed to be moved into the extended-care area of the home she was in, but this didn't happen. When Elinor went to find out why, she learned that Charlotte had sent in the appropriate government form to be moved (refusing to let anyone do it for her). On the form, Charlotte had written that she was self-sufficient. In fact, Elinor wrote Alex, "she had needed special nurses on two different occasions o.a.o. the Gov't keeps pushing new patients on the hospital without giving them more nurses and the four patients in Charlotte's area have to be selfdoing now; she can't walk without assistance and needs a wheelchair mostly."[25]

The government reply came back that Charlotte fit no guidelines. Now *that*, most citizens can attest, is a formidable obstacle. This was a battle tailor-made for Dr. Elinor F.E.

Black. Elinor learned that "if you are a millionaire, or there-abouts, the Gov't will not pay things for you, otherwise you are entirely in the Gov't hands and may do nothing on your own. This meant that Charlotte would be stashed in some Holding Facility until the Arbutus, where she has lived for the past 7 years, had room for her in the Extended Care area — seems the Gov't does not know what uncertainty and changing surroundings do to the elderly when they are ill and confused." Elinor wrote Alex, "I resolved to storm the ramparts."

In short order Elinor was able to report that Charlotte

> . . . picked up something lovely when I told her she would be going back to her "own nest'" and not to an unknown place. Later it was decreed that she could actually go back to her old room providing she would pay the $30/day she would have to pay for 3 practical nurses (in tot, not each) until they can give her a private room in the E.C. ward. Now, I think I done real good for me sister, but one never knows until one meets a minister nephew and his wife who think it very reprehensible that I should use my "profession, position, prestige and GALL" to do that for (go and get a cold beer, seems I ain't finished yet . . .) my sister when there were so many other people in her situation who had no one to help them. This kinda threw me o.a.o. I never thought of me as being a "gall-y" person.[26]

The minister nephew was Harold. He was happy for Charlotte but uncomfortable thinking Elinor had used "personal influence" to achieve her ends. That was pretty much the end of him. As Charlotte herself could have told Harold, anyone who questioned what Elinor did to protect or be with a loved one did so at his or her peril. Elinor wrote her nephew off as an "NDP radical" and broke another link between herself and her family.

Throughout 1977-78, as Charlotte began failing badly, Elinor's diary reads, "Wrote letters violently all day. I am provoked"; "more writing of letters"; "wrote letters frantically." It's as though time was running out to shore up what was slipping, correct what was wrong, reverse the trend. Elinor didn't neglect the details. When a grandniece gave her daughter an unusual name, Elinor took a moment to fire off a note to the new parents, "pointing out what they have done."[27]

Anger and heartbreak. Charlotte could no longer speak, although she understood what was said to her. One day Elinor received a letter. The stamp was stuck on crazily, and Charlotte's handwriting on the envelope was a wavering scrawl. When Elinor opened it, there was nothing inside.

Charlotte died in May 1979. Six months earlier, Elinor had tripped, broken her pelvis and left arm, and spent a month in hospital. By April she was off crutches, using a cane, and, defying her own unsteadiness and those who said Charlotte wouldn't remember her visit, she flew out to "hold Charlotte's hand" for awhile. Elinor did not return for the funeral. She told a young relative to arrange the service, adding, from the depths of her bitter loneliness, "It will be good practice for you!"[28]

Elinor's papers contain large stacks of affectionate, newsy letters from family members and many friends, letters dating through the end of the 1970s and into the 1980s. Many more friends were in Winnipeg, accessible by phone. But Elinor's pain came from knowing she no longer came first for anyone, she had no one left who came first for her. After Charlotte died, Elinor stopped keeping a diary.

Elinor returned to work but she was finding little solace there. Roulston had resigned, and in 1978 Dr. John Tyson became the new head. Tyson was a research scientist, an endocrinologist from Johns Hopkins. When Elinor learned of his appointment, she wrote, "Tyson our new prof! woe! woe!"[29] According to various colleagues, Elinor "just *bristled*" whenever she saw Tyson or heard anything about him.

Elinor just bet, she said, that Tyson would go in for "that in Vitro stuff"[30] while she was having to show fourth-year students where the urethra was. Elinor was deeply uneasy about what was yet to be named the new reproductive technologies (NRTs). She was also appalled at what she felt were fabulously expensive experiments to save increasingly tiny premature babies, to push back, one day at a time, the point at which a two-pound foetus was "viable" outside the womb. To Elinor it seemed like the only question being asked was, "We can do these fancy things, so why not?"[31]

Howard Taylor's report might have asked, had neonatology and NRTs been established fields in the 1960s, "Will these disciplines — because of the tremendous opportunity to conquer the mortality rates (of 750-gram preemies and embryonic emplants) — steal all the talented men?"

Meanwhile, Elinor felt, "the young doctors go to the country and have their first three mat. cases just pop out, then the next one sticks a bit and they do not know what to do so they phone a city Obstetrician who says if there is no OBS person there to phone the doctor who does the surgery in the community to come and do a Caesar."[32]

A few months before her death, Elinor was asked by students if it was all right to discharge a patient because the ultrasound showed no endometriosis. Elinor wrote Alex, "What did the pelvis feel like?" asks me; "Oh! I didn't do a pelvic on her!" comes from each one of them, so I went into my little homily and Miss Bloomfield, my British chief, who always said one had to do 1,000 P.V.'s before anyone could feel/find a mass smaller than a turnip — and they of course gave me the pitying look one gives old people not right in the head."[33]

Alex offered what comfort he could. Elinor wrote to him, and Molly, his wife, "Please excuse me! I didn't mean to blub all over Alex when I called this morning but every now and again, especially first thing in the A.M. I become so depressed and sorry for myself — I feel that Florence Nightingale really had something when she went to bed for 40 years and no one ever diagnosed her illness."[34] Alex wrote back, "I was struck by your mention that you feel depressed first thing in the morning for that is what I have noticed in the last two or three years. Existence seems pointless, the things to which one's time is devoted are so trivial, unnecessary, superfluous. . . . So you are not alone in feeling low and even tearful in the early hours."[35]

Elinor rallied. She taught a clinic two days before she died. On January 20, 1982, she wrote Alex, "As I was going to sleep last night, I wrote youse a long letter all about my first year in London and what fun I had. When I awakened this morning, the fluency had dissipated and now even my writing has gone all tiny. *Damn* the passing years!!"[36] The news arrived before the letter did; Elinor was gone. Her last words were of struggle and defiance. They were also, in evoking that first year in London, a reminder that she had realized a dream. She had gone to medical school, *press on*, she had gone to London, *press on*, she had shown them all. *No man shall place a limit in thy strength / Some feet will tread all heights now unattained / Why not thine own? Press on; Achieve!*

The first woman Member, the first woman Fellow, the first woman chair, the first woman president — Elinor Black achieved these for all Canadian women. Along the way she saw the CMA change the Ladies Program to the Spouses or Guest Program, the Manitoba Club close its side entrance and allow women through the front doors — and the numbers of female students in Canadian medical schools grow until women composed almost 50 percent of the enrollment.

She lived to see the pendulum beginning to swing back — toward a reduction in technologically governed labour and birth. In the 1950s, some of her colleagues had uttered warnings: "Doctors are becoming more and more and women are becoming less essential to labour";[37] and "Men became obsessed with [surgery] as more and more conditions proved amenable to surgical intervention."[38] By 1980, the rates of Caesarian sections and other interventions had become so high that the criticism could not be ignored.

In 1979, the *Lancet* published this observation from a frustrated contributer: "Sometimes I see the whole obstetric scene as a sort of angry triangle with doctor, midwife and patient confronting each other, and making contact only at the brief abrasive angles."[39] In 1980, *Maclean's* magazine published a critical look at the C-section rate, entitled, "Doctor's Choice, Mother's Trauma."[40] Some feminist health-care activists organized for change; some midwives and patients simply opted out of the triangle.

Elinor did not live to see a widespread adoption of her beliefs on hormone replacement therapy. *Ms.*, in a 1988 article entitled "The Estrogen Fix," quoted one doctor as asserting, "The consensus of doctors, the *worldwide* consensus, is that unless there is a counterindication, every menopausal woman should be given estrogen indefinitely to prevent osteoporosis and because of its other beneficial effects."[41] (Boy! one is tempted to react, you shoulda heard Elinor hammering on her casket.) *Ms.*, with its critical look at that assertion, added its protest and analysis to that of the many other women — and some men — who have carried on this particular battle.[42]

It's just as well, perhaps, that Elinor didn't live to see the end of obstetrical services and labour floors in some small-town hospitals. Women were still having babies, but the local doctors didn't feel confident enough about delivering them without the surgical and technological back-up that larger hospitals could provide if something went wrong. In 1986, the Ontario ombusdsman got involved in one case where the community demanded continued service. The subsequent report indicated that there was "no way to force doctors in private practice to do deliveries."[43]

One is glad, grateful, that Elinor did not live to see a news story that was picked up by the Canadian Press (CP) wire service on June 23, 1988. In another way, though, one longs for her to have taken up pen and paper, and in her orotund way delivered a barb so sharp . . .

The story, originating in Winnipeg, was this:

> A proposal by the President of the Manitoba Medical Association to make it easier for men than women to get into medical school has been given preliminary approval by Health Minister Don Orchard.
>
> Dr. Martin Thornington said recently he believes it would help get doctors into rural Manitoba where they are needed. He said roughly half the graduates of medical school in Manitoba are women, but they are reluctant to move out of Winnipeg into the country, where there is no day care and where their husbands might not find work.
>
> "It's not a popular issue, but I don't think there's any alternative," he said of a proposed quota that would favour men. Orchard said it was something the Faculty of Medicine at the University of Manitoba should consider.[44]

When Reverend James Uhrich looked out at the people gathered to mourn Elinor Black's death, he knew little, really, of the consuming passions and battles of her life. He had attempted a pastoral visit, when someone told him of Elinor's ill health and isolation, but he had been rather curtly dismissed. And yet, Uhrich must have understood a great deal in the short time he'd had to talk with those who knew Elinor. He spoke:

> We celebrate the life of Elinor Black.
> A life well-lived and useful . . .
> A life that has influenced countless other lives, gifted
> them, healed them, understood them,

and called them to account.
A perceptive and caustic humour
that gave occasion for thought as well as laughter.
A citizen of the world
as well as this city.
A respected professional, a tireless educator, a breaker of
new ground, a commanding and gracious presence . . .
The body that once cleared hurdles in such grand style has
finished its work.
The will that served her so well and which so many had
occasion to meet head on is at rest.

Four days after the service, the phone rang in Uhrich's office. The caller had just learned of Elinor's death. Sensing his great distress, Reverend Uhrich tried gently to convince the man to come in, or give his name so he could be visited. No, no, the caller said. He just needed to talk about her for awhile. He had loved her, and now she was gone and—he just needed to talk.

More people might have loved and admired Elinor Black than she knew. Perhaps she did not have to live with such a shell around her, with such loneliness after Gertrude died. Then again, perhaps she did. James Uhrich, in the memorial service, said it best: "The silences of her life that no one knew but her rest with her."

▼

EPILOGUE

▼

ON ONE OF MY RESEARCH TRIPS to Winnipeg, I jumped in a cab, eager to go and interview someone who had known and worked with Elinor Black. When the cab went past Kelvin High School, I recalled Elinor's *CMAJ* piece, "Thinking Back," and I leaned forward to ask the driver, who was elderly, how long the high school had been at that location and how far it really was, on foot, from Kennedy Street. He answered my questions, but, of course, wanted to know why I had asked. I told him a little about the biography and he mused, "I used to drive a Dr. Black. I don't know if her name was Elinor or not. Kind of a formidable old . . ."

I leaned forward again. How did he know her name, I asked. He didn't usually know the names of his fares, did he? "But that's just it," he said. "I remember her because she always told the dispatcher the same thing. You see, she always asked for a cab for Dr. Black but she thought the driver wouldn't be on the lookout for a woman. Some man, she said, would grab her cab, that had happened before, the driver would just assume . . ."

I can see that, I thought. "So what did she always say?" I was imagining that "my good fellow" tone. By now the cab was parked and I had learned the cabbie's name. Mr. Ryplanski turned and repeated from memory what the dispatcher liked to repeat to him, "I need a car to such and such an address. It's for Dr. Black. And tell the driver — Dr. Black is a woman."

Notes

Sources for the quotations at the opening of each chapter are given without a note number at the beginning of the notes for the chapter.

Much of the quoted material in this volume is taken from Elinor Black's papers, which are held privately by family members.

Chapter One: Family Players

Letter from Elinor Black to Frank Black, January 26, 1913.

1 Letter from Elinor Black to Dr. Alex Andison, March 9, 1981, Winnipeg.
2 Donald M. Black, M.D., "Francis Molison Black, 1870-1941" (unpublished), 1966, p. 22. Provincial Archives of Manitoba.
3 Frank Black, "Patrick Burns as I Knew Him," *Saturday Night* (March 27, 1937).
4 James H. Gray, *Red Lights on the Prairies* (Toronto: Macmillan of Canada, 1971), p. 140.
5 Ibid., pp. 141, 187.
6 Ibid., p. 186.
7 Donald Black, "Francis," p. 15.
8 Letter from Margaret Black to Frank Black, January 30, 1913.
9 Letter from Elinor Black and Margaret Black to Frank Black, May 18, 1913.
10 Isabelle M. Pagan first published *From Pioneer to Poet or The Twelve Great Gates: An Expansion of the Signs of the Zodiac Analysed* with the Theosophical Publishing House London Limited in 1911. The fifth and final edition was published in 1969 by Richard Clay Limited (The Chaucer Press), Bungay, Suffolk.
11 Letter from Frank Black to Elinor Black, Calgary, April 18, 1913.
12 Letters from Elinor Black to Frank Black, Christmas 1913; March 16, 1913.
13 Letter from Margaret Black and Elinor Black to Frank Black, May 18, 1913.
14 Letters from Elinor Black to Frank Black, Christmas 1913; January 26, 1913; March 5, 1913.
15 Letter from Elinor Black to Donald Black, Calgary, February 18, 1914.
16 Jessie A. McGeachy, M.D., "A Career in Obstetrics and Gynaecology," *Ontario Medical Review*, vol. 19 (1952):236.
17 Donald Black, "Francis," pp. 27-28.

18 Francis Marion Beynon, *Aleta Dey* (London: Virago Press, 1988), p. 163. *Aleta Dey* was first published in 1919 by C.W. Daniel Ltd., Great Britain.

19 On December 6, 1917, the Belgian relief vessel *Imo* collided with the French munitions carrier *Mont Blanc* in the narrowest part of Halifax Harbour. The munitions ship blew a mile high; over two and a half square kilometres of Halifax was levelled.

20 Harry Medovy, M.D., *A Vision Fulfilled: The Story of the Children's Hospital of Winnipeg, 1909-1973* (Winnipeg: Peguis Publishers Limited, 1979), pp. 21-22.

21 Elinor Black, "The Professor and His Wife," unpublished, p. 1. A reference in Elinor's diary indicates she finished the manuscript August 28, 1971. A copy of "Professor" is held in the Department of Archives and Special Collections, Elizabeth Dafoe Library, University of Manitoba.

22 Elinor Black, "Professor," p. 7.

23 Letter from Charlotte Black to Santa, November 24, 1913.

24 Letter from Elinor Black to Santa, undated, note in margin reads, "14 years old."

25 Charlotte Black to friend, undated. Original letter in the Department of Archives and Special Collections, Elizabeth Dafoe Library, University of Manitoba.

26 Elinor Black, "Thinking Back," *Canadian Medical Association Journal (CMAJ)*, vol. 105 (July 1971):143.

27 The poem, by John Oxenham, is reproduced as it was written in the autograph book. A slightly different version, entitled "Everymaid," can be found in *The Treasury of Christian Poetry*, compiled by Lorraine Eitel et al., (Old Tappan, New Jersey: Fleming H. Revell Company, 1982), p. 140.

28 Author unknown.

29 Letter from Elinor Black to Margaret Black, January 27, 1920.

30 Letter from Elinor Black to Frank and Margaret Black, Winnipeg, February 8, 1920.

31 Elinor Black, "Professor," p. 9.

32 Donald Black, "Francis," p. 33.

33 *Manitoba Free Press* (February 1, 1923):15.

34 Letter from Elinor Black to Alex Andison. Dated only "Mebbe the 31st October ending."

35 *Brown and Gold*, University of Manitoba Yearbook, 1930, p. 135.

Chapter Two: Rebellion and Escape

Winifred Holtby, *Women and a Changing Civilization* (London: John Lane, The Bodley Head Ltd., 1934), p. 114.

1 Ibid., p. 4

2 Barbara Angel and Michael Angel, *Charlotte Whitehead Ross* (Winnipeg: Peguis Publishers Ltd., 1982), p. 17

3 Howard M. Clarke, M.D., *Sex in Education: or, a Fair Chance for the Girls* (Boston: James R. Osgood and Company, 1873), pp. 83-84.

4 Ibid., p. 179.

5 Carlotta Hacker, *The Indomitable Lady Doctors* (Toronto: Clarke Irwin, 1974), p. 62.

6 C.M. Godfrey, "Origins of Medical Education of Women in Ontario," *Medical History*, vol. 17 (1973):90.

7 Hacker, *Indomitable*, pp. 63-64.

8 Ibid., pp. 64-65.

9 J.D. Adamson, M.D., "The Manitoba Medical College, 1883-1958," *The Manitoba Review*, vol. 38 (1958):469.

10 H.B. Chown, M.D., "The Story of the Medical College: 'Worship Great Men,'" *University of Manitoba Medical Journal (UMMJ)*, vol. 5 (December 1933):30.

11 Eva Mader MacDonald, M.D., and Elizabeth M. Webb, "A Survey of Women Physicians in Canada, 1883-1964," *CMAJ*, vol. 94 (1966):table 2.

12 Ruben Bellan, *Winnipeg First Century: An Economic History* (Winnipeg: Queenston House Publishing Co. Ltd., 1978), pp. 163, 178.

13 J.W. Chafe, *An Apple for the Teacher*, The Winnipeg School Division No. 1., 1967, p. 91.

14 Bellan, *Winnipeg*, p. 181.

15 Chafe, *Apple*, p. 92.

16 Letter from a friend, Edith, to Elinor Black, Toronto, January 31, 1945.

17 "The Records of the Life of Jesus," known in the Student Christian Movement (SCM) as "The Records," was a parallel arrangement of the Synoptic gospels, permitting comparative study of the words and actions of Jesus. SCM founder Dr. Henry Sharman prepared "The Records." For an historical overview of the SCM, see *This One Thing*, Prepared by a Group of Friends, Student Christian Movement of Canada (Toronto: Thistle Printing Ltd., 1959).

18 *This One Thing*, p. 11.

19 Letter from Margaret Howes to author, October 30, 1989.

20 Letter from Elinor Black to Mary Nickle, undated.

21 Margaret Howes, interviewed by author, September 30, 1989.

22 Letter from Margaret Black to Elinor Black, September 2, 1927.

23 Marjorie Bennett, M.D., interviewed by author, June 11, 1989.

24 "Maternal Mortality," *Manitoba Medical Bulletin*, no. 78 (1928):10.

25 Elinor Black, "The Department of Obstetrics and Gynaecology," *UMMJ*, vol. 51, no. 3. (1981).

26 Elinor Black, "Department," p. 108.

27 Ibid.

28 Injecting boiled milk to combat infection is mentioned in James R. Goodall, M.D., "Puerperal Infections," *CMAJ* (May 1930):696.

29 Hon. J.W. (Jack) Pickersgill, interviewed by author, November 4, 1988.

30 Elinor Black, "Department," p. 111.

31 Ibid., p. 112.

32 Letter from Jeannie Jackson to Elinor Black, June 3, 1930.

33 Medovy, *Vision*, p. 24.

34 Ibid., p. 32.

35 Letter from Elinor Black to Frank and Margaret Black, August 17, 1930.

36 Letter from Jeannie Jackson to Elinor Black, July 29, 1930.

37 Ibid., September 26, 1930.

38 Elinor Black, "Professor," pp. 16-17.

Chapter Three: Whirlwind

Elinor Black, "London Life: 1930-1931," unpublished memoir, p. 5; letter from Bernard Collings, M.D., to Elinor Black, March 12, 1932.

1 Elinor Black to Frank and Margaret Black, October 10, 1930.

2 Letter from Frank Black to Elinor Black, October 3, 1930.

3 Letter from Elinor Black to Frank and Margaret Black, October 16, 1930.

4 Elinor Black, "London," p. 2.

5 Notes from Isabel McGill, M.D., to author, undated.

6 Ibid.

7 Elinor Black, "London," p. 3.

8 Letter from Elinor Black to Isabel McGill, M.D., May 13, 1949.

9 Letter from Isabel McGill, M.D., to author, May 24, 1989.

10 Elinor Black, "London," p. 4.

11 Letter from Elinor Black to Frank and Margaret Black, January 18, 1931.

12 Ibid.

13 Letters from Jeannie Jackson to Elinor Black, February 1, 1931; February 13, 1931; February 24, 1931; April 2, 1931.

14 Letter from Elinor Black to Frank and Margaret Black, January 25, 1931.

15 Elinor Black, "London," p. 5.

16 Ibid.

17 Letter from Frank Black to Elinor Black, Kelowna, May 24, 1931.

18 Letter from Jeannie Jackson to Elinor Black, April 2, 1931.

19 Letters from Frank Black to Elinor Black, Kelowna, May 3, 1931; May 5, 1931.

20 Letter from Frank Black to Elinor Black, February 2, 1931.

21 Ibid., May 24, 1931.

22 Letter from Elinor Black to Frank and Margaret Black, May 20, 1931.

23 Note written by Elinor Black, undated.

24 "Should Women Earn Pin Money?" *Maclean's* (April 1, 1930):60.

25 *Montreal Daily Star* (January 3, 1930):21.

26 Elinor Black, "Professor," p. 18.

27 Letter from Elinor Black to Margaret and Frank Black, April 38, 1931.

28 Ibid.

29 Letter from Elinor Black to Margaret and Frank Black, May 20, 1931.

30 Letter from A.N. MacLeod, M.D., to Elinor Black, February 5, 1931.

31 Letter from Elinor Black to Margaret and Frank Black, May 20, 1931.

Chapter Four: Struggle

Arianna Stassinopoulos, *The Gods of Greece* (McClelland and Stewart, Toronto, 1983), p. 140; Elinor Black, "Professor," p. 22.

1 Letter from J.S. Turner to Frank Black, Winnipeg, June 27, 1931.

2 Letter from Frank Black to Elinor Black, June 29, 1931.

3 Elinor Black, "Professor," p. 20.

4 Ibid., p. 21.

5 Letter from Elinor Black to Frank Black, July 5, 1931.

6 Elinor Black, "Professor," p. 36.

7 Ibid., p. 28; p. 27.

8 *Winnipeg Free Press* (April 3, 1933):11.

9 Jane Seaborne (formerly Bessie Pickersgill), interviewed by author, June 30, 1989.

10 Elinor Black, "A Pi Phi Doctor," *The May Arrow*, a magazine published by the Phi Beta Phi Fraternity (May 1936):201.

11 *Winnipeg Free Press* (April 3, 1933):11.

12 Minutes of Special Executive meeting of the Winnipeg Medical Society, December 10, 1931.

13 Elinor Black, "Professor," pp. 23-24.
14 Letter from Bernard Collings, M.D., to Elinor Black, December 18, 1931.
15 Letter from Sir Howard d'Egville to Elinor Black, December 24, 1931.
16 Letter from Bernard Collings, M.D., to Elinor Black, March 12, 1932.
17 *Brown and Gold*, University of Manitoba Yearbook, 1930, pp. 260-261.
18 Elinor Black, "London," p. 7.
19 Elinor Black, "Professor," pp. 29-30.
20 Grace Schell (nee Cameron), interviewed by author, October 2, 1990.
21 Letter from Elinor Black to Charlotte Black, May 3, 1932.
22 Letter from Bernard Collings, M.D., to Elinor Black, May 18, 1932.
23 Ibid.
24 Holtby, *Women*, pp. 132-133.
25 Ibid., p. 132.
26 Letter from Elinor Black to Charlotte Black, October 12, 1932.
27 Letter from Bernard Collings, M.D., to Elinor Black, March 22, 1936.
28 Letter from Elinor Black to Charlotte Black, May 5, 1932.
29 Letter from Elinor Black to Frank Black, November 29, 1932.
30 Letter from Elinor Black to Charlotte Black, May 5, 1932.
31 Ibid.
32 Ibid., August 6, 1932.
33 Ibid.
34 Letter from Isabel McGill, M.D., to Elinor Black, undated.
35 Letter from Elinor Black to Charlotte Black, March 25, 1932.
36 Minutes of the Winnipeg Medical Society meeting, November 18, 1932.
37 Ibid., December 16, 1932; January 20, 1933.
38 Letter from Elinor Black to Charlotte Black, August 6, 1932.
39 *The Manitoba Reports*, 1925-26, vol. 35, p. 300.
40 Ibid.
41 *Western Weekly Reports*, vol. 3 (1925):100.
42 Ibid., vol. 1 (1925):889.
43 Goodall, "Puerperal Infections," p. 694.
44 W.A. Dafoe, M.D., "The Types and Treatment of Abortions," *CMAJ* (June 1930):794.
45 Jean M. Dunmire, "The Winnipeg Birth Control Society in the 1930s: The Social Reform Lobby for a Healthy Birth Controlled World," unpublished paper, April 28, 1988, p. 5; p. 11. Provincial Archives of Manitoba.
46 Helen MacMurchy, M.D., *Sterilization? Birth Control?* (Toronto: The Macmillan Company of Canada Ltd., 1934), p. 24; p. 4.

47 Ibid., pp. 38-39.
48 Dunmire, "Winnipeg Birth Control," p. 18.
49 MacMurchy, *Sterilization?*, p. 124.
50 Letter from Elinor Black to Charlotte Black, March 25, 1933.
51 Ibid., April 13, 1933.
52 T. Glen Hamilton, *Intention and Survival* (Toronto: The Macmillan Company of Canada Ltd., 1942).
53 Ross Mitchell, M.D., *Medicine in Manitoba: The Story of its Beginnings* (Winnipeg: Manitoba Medical Assocation, 1955), p. 117. See also Margaret Lillian Hamilton, *Is Survival a Fact?* (London: Psychic Press Ltd., 1969), pp. 42-45.
54 Mitchell, *Medicine in Manitoba*, p. 117.
55 Letter from Elinor Black to Alex Andison, M.D., July 31, 1977.
56 Minutes of the Winnipeg Medical Society meeting, February 17, 1933 (emphasis mine).
57 The agreement between the Winnipeg Medical Society and the City of Winnipeg was signed May 8, 1934. The document is held by the City of Winnipeg Archives and Records Control. See also "Survey of Illness amongst Unemployed in the City of Winnipeg," *Manitoba Medical Association Review (MMAR)* (February 1937):25-26; and C.E. Corrigan, M.D., "Sixty Years of Medicine in Manitoba," *UMUJ*, vol. 44 (1974):12.
58 Corrigan, "Sixty Years," pp. 12-13.
59 Letter from Frank Black to Elinor Black, undated.
60 *Blue and White*, University of Manitoba Nurses' Yearbook, 1930, p. 55.
61 Letter from Elinor Black to Gertrude Rutherford, May 17, 1959.
62 Letter from Frank Black to Elinor Black, May 30, 1934.
63 Ibid., Sidney, British Columbia, February 18, 1935.
64 Ibid., February 20, 1935.
65 Ibid., February 18, 1935.

Chapter Five: Getting the "M"

Elinor Black, "Department," p. 110.
1 Elinor Black, "A Journey from Heidelburg to Prague in 1937," unpublished story/memoir, undated, p. 1.
2 Elinor Black, speech to the University of Manitoba's Women's Club, February 10, 1965.
3 Elinor Black, "Professor," p. 42.
4 Ibid., p. 43.
5 Bennett interview.

6 Cook's itinerary pamphlet, 1937.

7 Ibid.

8 Elinor Black, "Journey," p. 1.

9 Elinor Black, "Professor," p. 45.

10 Elinor Black, "How I Came to Know Annie French Rhead," unpublished story/memoir, undated, pp. 3-4.

11 Brian Best, M.D., interviewed by author, September 8, 1988.

12 "The South London Hospital for Women and Children," published by the Amenity Fund, March 1966, pp. 10-11. In a letter to the author dated January 20, 1989, Dr. Margaret Louden reported that, to her knowledge, the identities of the donors has not been revealed to date.

13 Letter from Margaret Louden, M.D., to Patricia Want, Royal College of Obstetricians and Gynaecologists (RCOG), September 28, 1988.

14 RCOG, Instructions to Examiners, Membership, February 1948.

15 Elinor Black, Obstetrical and Gynaecological Case Records, certified by D.S. MacKay, M.D., November 8, 1937. Case 11; Case 26; Case 27.

16 Ibid., Case 30.

17 Ibid., Case 27.

18 Ibid., Introduction, "The Routine Care of Pregnant Patients in the Antenatal Period and in Hospital."

19 "Maternal Mortality," p. 9.

20 "News Items," MMAR (October 1937):188.

21 Ross Mitchell, M.D., "Maternity Hospitals of Greater Winnipeg," Manitoba Medical Review (MMR), vol. 26 (May 1946):274-277.

22 Elinor Black, Case Records, Case 3.

23 Ibid., Section: "Streptococcal Puerperal Sepsis Treated with Animal Serum and Normal Human Blood Serum Transfusions."

24 Ibid.

25 Letter to Elinor Black, June 20, 1938, 114 Harley Street, signature illegible.

26 Hacker, Indomitable, p. 3.

27 Mrs. Harry Medovy, interviewed by author, June 1, 1989.

Chapter Six: Heartbreak and Loss

Thomas Carlyle, *Past and Present*, book 3, chapter 11 (London: J.M. Dent and Sons, Ltd., 1970), p. 190.

1 Clipping in Elinor's papers marked *Free Press*, no other reference. "Pi Phi Personalities," *The May Arrow* (1938):330, makes the same statement.

2 Alice Harriet Parsons, "Careers or Marriage?" *Canadian Home Journal (CHJ)* (June 1938):26, 63, 64.

3 *CHJ* (May 1938):3.

4 Ibid. (June 1938):64.

5 "Women in Medicine," *The Canadian Doctor* (April 1936):36-37. Article is signed only, "Say Men."

6 Steven M. Spencer, "Do Women Make Good Doctors?" *Saturday Evening Post* (November 13, 1948):15-17; 134-37; 141.

7 "Women in Medicine," p. 36.

8 Letter from friend to Elinor Black.

9 Letter from Orville M.M. Kay to Elinor Black, dated 11-2-38.

10 Margaret Lawrence Greene, *The School of Femininity: A Book for and about Women as They Are Interpreted through Feminine Writers of Yesterday and Today* (Toronto: Musson Book Company, 1972), p. 146. Lawrence Greene is quoting writer Olive Schreiner. Elinor had the 1936 edition of Lawrence Greene's book.

11 Letter from Elinor Black to Charlotte Black, April 29, 1939.

12 Bennett interview.

13 Margaret Georgina Todd, *The Life of Sophia Jex-Blake* (London: Macmillan and Company Ltd., 1918), p. 70.

14 Seaborne interview.

15 Letter from Bernard Collings, M.D., to Elinor Black, April 26, 1939.

16 Letter from Elinor Black to Charlotte Black, May 19, 1939.

17 Ibid., May 31, 1939.

18 Ibid., May 8, 1939.

19 Ibid., May 19, 1939.

20 Ibid., April 29, 1939.

21 Letter from Charlotte Black to Elinor Black, November 13, 1940.

22 Letter from Frank Black to Elinor Black, Vancouver, January 17, 1940.

23 Ibid., February 18, 1940.

24 *Winnipeg Free Press* (February 29, 1941):13; *Winnipeg Tribune* (February 20, 1941).

25 Letter from Margaret Scoular Black to Elinor Black, Hillview, April 28, 1941.

26 Letter from E. Mary Magill, M.D., to Elinor Black, Kent, April 28, 1941.

27 Letter from Margaret Louden, M.D., to author, January 20, 1989.

28 Vera Brittain, *Testament of Friendship* (London: Fontana, 1981), p. 352.

29 "First Fifty Years, 1895-1945: The Training and Work of Women Employed in the Service of the United Church of Canada" (Toronto: The United Church of Canada, n.d.), p. 31.

30 Letter from Harriet M. Perry, M.D., to Elinor Black, Winnipeg, January 9, 1945.

31 Letters from Edith to Elinor Black, January 2, 1945; January 23, 1945.

32 Letter from Charlotte Black to Elinor Black, May 20, 1945.

33 Letter from Connie Lethbridge to Elinor Black, July 25, 1945.

34 Letter from E. Mary Magill, M.D., to Elinor Black, Kent, November 11, 1944.

35 Unidentified news clipping, June 27, 1959.

36 Letter from Jane Seaborne to author, January 8, 1989.

37 "Successful in a Man's World," *Vancouver Daily Province* (October 7, 1944):8.

38 The news clipping headline, "Canadian Medical Men Gather in Winnipeg," and accompanying photographs are undated but refer to a Canadian Medical Association conference held in Winnipeg June 23-27, 1941.

39 *MMR*, vol. 24 (October 1944):271.

40 W.G. Cosbie, M.D., *The History of the Society of Obstetricians and Gynaecologists of Canada, 1944-1966*, published by the Society, 1967, p. 9.

41 J. Robert Willson, M.D., and Else Reid Carrington, M.D., *Obstetrics and Gynecology*, seventh edition (St. Louis: The C.V. Mosby Company, 1983), p. 51.

42 David B. Stewart, M.D., interviewed by author, September 8, 1988.

43 Cynthia Draper, interviewed by author, September 12, 1988.

44 Letter from Elinor Black to Gertrude Rutherford, September 1, 1958.

Chapter Seven: The Maternity Pavilion

Letter from Otto Schmidt, M.D., to Elinor Black, June 1, 1949.

1 Letter from Elinor Black to Alex Andison, M.D., Winnipeg, May 24, 1968.

2 Letter from Elinor Black to Isabel McGill, M.D., Winnipeg, February 17, 1950.

3 James Mitchell, M.D., interviewed by author, September 13, 1988.

4 Elinor Black, "Department," p. 105.

5 Otto Schmidt, M.D., interviewed by author, July 1989.

6 A.T. Cameron, M.D., "The Friedman Pregnancy Test," *MMR* (September 1944):255.

7 Elinor Black, "Not So Long Ago," *UMMJ*, vol. 45 (1975):56.

8 Medovy, *Vision*, p. 67.

9 Ibid., pp. 67-68.

10 *MMR*, vol. 24 (March 1944):68.

11 Ibid., vol. 25 (January 1945):30; vol. 25 (February 1945); vol. 25 (August 1945).

12 M. Sidney Margolese, M.D., "The Diagnosis and Treatment of the Climacteric," *MMR*, vol. 24 (April 1944):105.

13 Elinor Black, "The Use of Testosterone Propionate in Gynaecology," *CMAJ* (August 1942):124.

14 Ibid., pp. 124-128.

15 Elinor Black, "The Uses and Abuses of Endocrine Therapy," *MMR*, vol. 25 (November 1945):475-479.

16 David B. Steward, M.D., interviewed by author, September 8, 1988.

17 Elinor Black, "Endocrine Therapy," p. 475.

18 Elinor Black, "Professor," p. 67.

19 Letter from Elinor Black to Jack Pickersgill, January 5, 1949.

20 Elinor Black's trip diary, December 7, 1948; March 18, 1949; March 15, 1949; March 18, 1949.

21 Ibid., March 17, 1949.

22 Elinor Black, "The Blue Grass Disaster," unpublished memoir/story, undated.

23 Letter from Elinor Black to Isabel McGill, M.D., May 13, 1949.

24 Ibid., S.S. *Britannia*, May 30, 1949.

25 Ibid., Stockholm, June 1, 1949.

26 Ibid.

27 Ibid., June 4, 1949.

28 Ibid., June 10, 1949.

29 Ibid., June 4, 1949.

30 Ibid., June 10, 1949.

31 Ibid.

32 Ibid., Cumberland Hotel, June 28, 1949.

33 Ibid.

34 Ibid., Southampton, July 7, 1949.

35 Letters from Isabel McGill, M.D., to Elinor Black, May 4, 1949; May 10, 1949.

36 Letter from Elinor Black to Isabel McGill, M.D., July 16, 1949.

37 Ibid., Mansonville, August 10, 1949.

38 Letter from Eva Macfarlane to Elinor Black, May 27, 1952.

39 Letter from Elinor Black to Gertrude Rutherford, May 19, 1950.

40 Letter from Elinor Black to Isabel McGill, M.D., Mansonville, August 10, 1949.

41 Notes from Isabel McGill, M.D., to author, undated.

42 Letter from Elinor Black to Isabel McGill, M.D., August 27, 1949.

43 Ibid., Winnipeg, September 23, 1949; undated.

44 Elinor Black, "Department," p. 106.

45 Letter from David Stewart, M.D., to Elinor Black, Aberdeen, January 20, 1950.

46 Letter from Elinor Black to Isabel McGill, M.D., Winnipeg, September 23, 1949.

47 Letter from Elinor Black to Gertrude Rutherford, April 30, 1950.

48 Letter from Elinor Black to Isabel McGill, M.D., Winnipeg, September 23, 1949.

49 The newspapers are the *Winnipeg Tribune*, the *Winnipeg Free Press*, the *Toronto Star*, the *Globe and Mail*, the *Nelson Daily News*, the *Hamilton Free Press*, the *Regina Leader-Post*, the *Edmonton Journal* and *Le courrier d'eastview*. The *Saturday Night* mention is April 4, 1950, p. 27.

50 Letter from Elinor Black to Isabel McGill, M.D., Winnipeg, February 17, 1950.

51 Ibid.

52 Elinor Black, "Professor," p. 70.

53 Letter from Elinor Black to Isabel McGill, M.D., Winnipeg, March 26, 1950.

54 Ibid., February 17, 1950.

Chapter Eight: The Flood!

"Close-Up," Canadian Broadcasting Corporation (CBC) Television, November 3, 1957.

1 W.D. Hurst, "The Red River Flood of 1950," paper read before the Historical and Scientific Society of Manitoba, series 3, no. 12, 1957, p. 57.

2 Ralph Allen, "You Can't Lick a River That Won't Fight Back," *Maclean's* (July 1, 1950):7.

3 Hurst, "Flood," p. 76

4 Ron Tuckwell, "Morris Member Stresses Flood Danger in Legislature," *The Morris Herald* (April 20, 1950).

5 Letter from Elinor Black to Gertrude Rutherford, April 30, 1950.

6 Ibid., May 6, 1950.

7 *The Morris Herald* (June 15, 1950):1.

8 Frank Rasky, *Great Canadian Disasters* (Toronto: Longmans Green and Company, 1961), pp. 169-172.

9 "Black Friday" was May 5, 1950. The use of "black" or "dark" as equivalent to "negative" or in connection with natural or financial disasters reflects a racial prejudice.

10 Hurst, "Flood," p. 75.

11 Rasky, *Disasters*, p. 181.

12 *Maclean's*, editorial (July 15, 1950).

13 Rasky, *Disasters*, p. 182.

14 Ibid., p. 179.

15 Hurst, "Flood," p. 71.

16 Rasky, *Disasters*, p. 167.

17 *Winnipeg Free Press* (May 7, 1950):1.

18 Elinor Black, "Department," p. 106.

19 Ibid.

20 Elinor Black, "The Maternity Pavilion," *Winnipeg Free Press* (May 3, 1952):21.

21 Letter from Elinor Black to Gertrude Rutherford, May 6, 1950.

22 Ibid.

23 Ibid., May 9, 1950.

24 "Close-Up," November 3, 1957.

25 Letter from Elinor Black to Gertrude Rutherford, May 6, 1950.

26 Ibid.

27 Ibid., May 7, 1950.

28 Ibid., May 8, 1950; May 16, 1950.

29 Ibid., May 8, 1950.

30 Ibid., May 9, 1950.

31 Ibid., May 10, 1950. Elinor often used "we" for "I" when she wrote to Gertrude, as in "we bin running."

32 Hurst, "Flood," p. 77.

33 Here again, the use of "black" as equivalent to "negative" reflects a racial prejudice.

34 Hurst, "Flood," pp. 77-78.

35 Allen, "Can't Lick," p. 7.

36 Letter from Elinor Black to Gertrude Rutherford, May 12, 1950.

37 Ibid., May 13, 1950.

38 Ibid., May 14, 1950.

39 Hurst, "Flood," p. 78.

40 Letter from Elinor Black to Gertrude Rutherford, May 16, 1950.

41 Ibid., May 19, 1950.

42 Ibid., May 16, 1950.

43 Ibid., May 19, 1950.

44 Ibid., May 17, 1950.

45 Hurst, "Flood," p. 78.

46 Letter from Elinor Black to Gertrude Rutherford, May 19, 1950.

47 J.W. Pickersgill, *My Years with Louis St. Laurent* (Toronto: University of Toronto Press, 1975), pp. 108-110.

48 Jack Pickersgill interview.

49 Rasky, *Disasters*, p. 187.
50 Jack Pickersgill interview.
51 Rasky, *Disasters*, p. 187.
52 Letter from Elinor Black to Gertrude Rutherford, May 21, 1950.
53 Ibid., May 17, 1950.

Chapter Nine: Recognition

Marie Storrie, M.D., interviewed by author, April 23, 1988; letter from Ina
    Broadfoot to Elinor Black, November 10, 1951.
 1 Letter from Doris Saunders to Elinor Black, November 14, 1951.
 2 Letter from May to Elinor Black, Glasgow, December 8, 1951.
 3 Letter from David Stewart, M.D., to Elinor Black, Aberdeen, January
    11, 1952.
 4 Chas. V. Neal, Jr., "A Girl Should Work before Marriage," *Winnipeg
    Free Press* (July 26, 1958):18.
 5 Betty Stapleton, "Need Give and Take when Doctors Hitch in Double
    Harness," *Toronto Daily Star* (July 6, 1964):35-38.
 6 Letter from Jan Macdonald to Elinor Black, December 16, 1951.
 7 Letter from Charlotte Black to Elinor Black, dated only "Wednesday
    evening."
 8 Letter from Edie to Elinor Black, undated.
 9 MacDonald and Webb, "Survey." Table 3 shows that the percentage of
    women surgeons in Canada in 1964 was 1.2.
10 Perri Klass, M.D., *A Not Entirely Benign Procedure* (New York: Signet,
    1987), pp. 92-95.
11 Best interview.
12 Rhinehart Friesen, M.D., interviewed by author, April 26, 1988.
13 W.J. Friesen, M.D., interviewed by author, April 26, 1988.
14 *British Medical Journal*, July 9, 1955, p. 112.
15 Letter from Elinor Black to Gertrude Rutherford, June 8, 1950.
16 A. Naimark, M.D., interviewed by author, September 15, 1988.
17 Patient and friend of Elinor Black, name withheld, interviewed by
    author, June 1989.
18 Alex Andison, M.D., after-dinner speech at Elinor Black's retirement
    dinner, November 13, 1964.
19 Letter from A.H.S. Gillson to Elinor Black, November 8, 1951.
20 Letter from F.W. Crawford to Elinor Black, June 2, 1950.
21 Letter from David Stewart, M.D., to Elinor Black, Aberdeen, January
    11, 1952.
22 Letter from A.D. Kelly, M.D., to Elinor Black, Toronto, November 30,
    1951.

23 Letter from Ina Broadfoot to Elinor Black, November 10, 1951.

24 Letter from Jan Macdonald to Elinor Black, December 16, 1951.

25 Letter from Lillias C.-MacIntyre, M.D., to Elinor Black, December 8, 1951.

26 Letter from A. Kiernan to Elinor Black, March 14, 1951.

27 Letter from John Zack, M.D., to Elinor Black, December 28, 1953.

28 Elinor Black, "Reply to a Toast, CMA Mtg circa 1952," notes.

29 Letter from W.R. Feasby, M.D., editor of *Modern Medicine of Canada*, Toronto, to Elinor Black, February 28, 1955.

30 "Dean of Medicine Spikes Taboos on Women Doctors," February 25, 1956, newspaper clipping in Elinor Black's papers.

31 Letter from W.F. Tisdale, M.D., to Elinor Black, January 19, 1954.

32 Elinor Black attached a copy of her response to Dr. Tisdale's letter.

33 *Journal of the American Medical Women's Association*, October 1952, p. 394.

34 Ibid., p. 393.

35 Letter from Elinor Black to Gertrude Rutherford, June 21, 1950.

36 Elinor Black, "Infertility," paper presented to the 46th Annual Meeting, College of Physicans and Surgeons of Saskatchewan, CMA Division, 1953.

37 Elinor Black, "Some Sociological Aspects of Sterilization," paper read at the American College of Obstetricians and Gynecologists, District 6, 10th Annual Conference on Obstetric, Gynecologic and Neonatal Nursing, Winnipeg, October 6, 1969.

38 Andison, after-dinner speech.

39 Elinor Black, review, *Modern Medicine of Canada*, June 1954, pp. 118-119.

40 Alex Andison, M.D., interviewed by author, August 10, 1988.

41 Mitchell interview. Elinor Black's submission to the Winnipeg General Hospital Annual Report in 1963, the year before she retired, gives a C-section rate of 4.27 percent.

42 Elinor Black, "Thinking Back," *CMAJ* (July 24, 1971):144.

43 Andison interview, August 10, 1988.

44 Comrie McCawley, M.D., interviewed by author, June 1989.

45 Letter from Elinor Black to Gertrude Rutherford, June 8, 1950.

46 Grantly Dick-Read, M.D., wrote about a related issue in *Childbirth without Fear*, 5th edition (New York: Harper and Row, 1984). Dick-Read noted that rates of forceps deliveries for private patients were much higher than for "clinic" patients. He wrote, "Why was the forceps rate of the white, brown, and black clinic population so much

lower than for white private patients whose fees were higher?" (p. 309). Elinor's trip diary, January 4, 1949, notes that in one hospital, 36 percent of private patients were diagnosed as having endometriosis compared to eight percent of public patients.

47 Elinor Black, "Symposium on Caesarian Section," *MMR*, vol. 30 (1950):355-356.

48 Jean McFarlane, M.D., interviewed by author, September 12, 1988.

49 Elinor Black, "The Treatment of Dysmenorrhoea with Phenylbutazone," *CMAJ*, vol. 79 (November 1, 1958):752.

50 *CMAJ*, vol. 74 (June 1, 1956):48-49.

51 Elinor Black, "Gynaecological Endocrinology," *MMR*, vol. 45 (June/July 1965):344.

52 Elinor Black, "Endometriosis," paper given to the Hamilton Academy of Medicine, January 1962, pp. 11-12.

53 Elinor Black, address to the British Congress of Obstetrics and Gynaecology, Cardiff, 1959.

54 Elinor Black, "The Menopause," the *Globe and Mail* (December 12, 1956):14.

55 Statistics table in *MMAR* (February 1937):28.

56 Elinor Black, "Foreword," *Modern Medicine of Canada* (March 1952):28.

57 Elinor Black, "The Menopause," p. 14.

58 Schmidt interview.

59 See, Kathleen McDonnell, ed., *Adverse Effects: Women and the Pharmaceutical Industry* (Toronto: The Women's Press, 1986); *D.E.S.: An Uncertain Legacy*, National Film Board of Canada, Studio D, 1985; Gena Corea, *The Hidden Malpractice: How American Medicine Mistreats Women* (New York: Harper and Row, 1985); Ruth Hubbard et al., eds., *Women Look at Biology Looking at Women* (Cambridge, Massachusetts: Schenkman Publishing Co., 1979); Kathryn Strother Ratcliff, ed., *Healing Technology: Feminist Perspectives* (Ann Arbor: The University of Michigan Press, 1989); Ellen Lewin and Virginia Olesen, eds., *Women, Health and Healing: Toward a New Perspective* (New York: Tavistock Publications, 1985); Boston Women's Health Collective, *The New Our Bodies, Ourselves* (New York: Simon and Schuster, Inc., 1984).

60 Letter from Elinor Black to Dr. S. Vaisrub, editor, *MMR*, Winnipeg, November 9, 1957.

61 Dick-Read, *Childbirth*, p. xx. The preface originally appeared in the 1933 edition, entitled *Natural Childbirth* (London: Heinemann).

62 The 1944 edition, entitled *Childbirth without Fear*, was published by Harper and Bros., New York.

63 June Callwood, "Painless Childbirth — Sometimes," *Maclean's*, (July 15, 1950):50.

64 "Close-Up," CBC Television, November 3, 1957.

65 Dorothy Guest, interviewed by author, June 7, 1989.

66 Letters from "an old patient" to Elinor Black, Fort William, Ontario, November 4, 1957; George G. Kerster, M.D. to Elinor Black, Vancouver, November 13, 1957; Elsie Wilson to Elinor Black, November 5, 1957; May Smith to Elinor Black, Montreal, dated only "Tuesday evening"; Patrick Watson to Elinor Black, Toronto, November 5, 1957.

67 Letters from Gwen Neale to Elinor Black, dated only "6:30 a.m. April 22nd"; Janie Merle McEachen to Elinor Black, Winnipeg, November 27, 1951; Ida B. to Elinor Black, December 24, 1951.

68 Letter from Elinor Black to Edith, Barrie, July 24, 1957.

69 Letter from Mrs. Parker to Elinor Black, Winnipeg, August 15, 1957.

70 *Safeguarding Motherhood: The Winnipeg General Hospital Maternity Wards 1888-1950*, published by the Board of Trustees of the Winnipeg General Hospital, p. 7.

71 Mrs. Howcroft, interviewed by author, June 8, 1989; May Clarke, interviewed by author, June 8, 1989.

72 Letters from Eva Macfarlane to Elinor Black, July 1, 1957; July 23, 1957.

73 Letter from Mrs. Parker to Elinor Black, August 15, 1957.

Chapter Ten: Around the World — and Back

Letters from Elinor Black to Gertrude Rutherford, August 4, 1958; Nairobi, March 3, 1959.

1 Elinor Black, "Professor," p. 99.

2 Letter from Jean McFarlane, M.D., to Elinor Black, July 26, 1956.

3 Letter from Sir Charles Read, M.D., to Elinor Black, March 12, 1957.

4 Letter from J.W. Pickersgill to the Heads of Canadian Missions Abroad, Ottawa, July 3, 1958.

5 Letters from Elinor Black to Gertrude Rutherford, July 24, 1958; Vancouver, July 29, 1958.

6 Ibid., Seattle, August 1, 1958.

7 Ibid., August 4, 1958.

8 Ibid., August 27, 1958.

9 Ibid., August 18, 1958.

10 Ibid., November 27, 1958.

11 Ibid., Genoa, April 5, 1959.

12 Ibid., Cambridge, May 22, 1959.

13 Letter from Elinor Black to Isabel McGill, M.D., Vancouver, December 26, 1949.
14 Letters from Elinor Black to Gertrude Rutherford, Beppu, September 6, 1958; December 10, 1958.
15 Ibid., November 3, 1958.
16 Elinor Black, "The Shark-Fishing Episode off the Great Barrier Reef," memoir/story, unpublished, undated, p. 1.
17 Letter from Elinor Black to Gertrude Rutherford, October 22, 1958.
18 Elinor Black, "Shark," p. 4.
19 Ibid.
20 *Brown and Gold*, University of Manitoba Yearbook, 1930, p. 135.
21 Letter from Elinor Black to Gertrude Rutherford, October 22, 1958.
22 Elinor Black, "Shark," p. 5.
23 Ibid., p. 6.
24 McFarlane interview.
25 Letter from Elinor Black to Gertrude Rutherford, Edinburgh, July 25, 1959.

Chapter Eleven: A Losing Battle

Comrie McCawley, M.D., interviewed by author, June 1989.
1 Elinor Black, "Department," p. 106.
2 McFarlane interview.
3 Letter from Elinor Black to Gertrude Rutherford, November 8, 1959.
4 Elinor Black, pocket diary, February 1, 1960.
5 Letter from Connie Lethbridge to Elinor Black, January 26, 1960.
6 John Lindsay, M.D., interviewed by author, June 4, 1989.
7 Elinor Black, pocket diary, January 24, 1960; January 21, 1960.
8 Ibid., July 20, 1960; August 6, 1960; August 27, 1960.
9 Letter from Gertrude Rutherford to Elinor Black, January 12, 1962.
10 Elinor Black, pocket diary, February 27, 1962.
11 Letter from Elinor Black to K. Harriet Christie, Principal, United Church Training School, February 28, 1962.
12 *Globe and Mail* (March 16, 1961); *Toronto Star* (March 1, 1962).
13 Unidentified clipping sent to Elinor Black in letter from Laura K. Pelton, Toronto, September 26, 1962.
14 Letter from Mary Macdougall to Eva Macfarlane, Angola, March 19, 1962; letter passed on to Elinor Black; letter from Ruth Arndt to Elinor Black, Pretoria, undated; letter from Gwen Kidd to Elinor Black, Littlehampton, April 30, 1962; letter from Helen Ellis to Elinor Black, Chesire, March 6; letter from Jan Macdonald to Elinor Black, Dorset,

March 9; letter from Constance Chappell to Elinor Black, Toronto,
Friday, March 2; letter from Helen Ellis to Elinor Black, Cheshire,
March 6; letter from Jan Macdonald to Elinor Black, Dorset, March 9;
letter from Eva Macfarlane to Elinor Black, March 11, 1962; letter from
Gwen Kidd to Elinor Black, Littlehampton, April 30, 1962.

15 Elinor Black, "Professor," p. 106.

16 Elinor Black, pocket diary, October 31, 1960.

17 Ibid., October 28, 1961.

18 Ibid., May 25, 1964.

19 McCawley interview.

20 Clarke interview.

21 Ibid.

22 Mary Schutte, interviewed by author, June 11, 1989; letter from Elinor
Black to Alex Andison, January 5, 1975.

23 Elinor Black, address to the University Women's Club of Winnipeg,
February 10, 1965.

24 Ibid.

25 Letter from Gwen Kidd to Elinor Black, February 17, 1964.

26 Greene, *School*.

27 Elinor Black, presidential address to the Society of Obstetricians and
Gynaecologists of Canada, St. Adele, Quebec, June 17, 1961. Published
in *CMAJ*, vol. 85 (October 21, 1961):940-942.

28 *Financial Post* (November 18, 1961):9.

29 Letter from H.B. Atlee, M.D., to Elinor Black, Halifax, October 10,
1961.

30 Letter from S. McClatchie, M.D., to Elinor Black, Vancouver, November 22.

31 Letter from L.G. Bell, M.D., to H.H. Saunderson, May 9, 1961.

32 Letter from Elinor Black to L.G. Bell, M.D., September 17, 1960.

33 Letter from C.A. Woolever, M.D.

34 Letter from O.A. Schmidt to Elinor Black, Winnipeg, May 25, 1961.

35 Letter from David B. Stewart, M.D., to Elinor Black, May 26, 1964.

36 Howard C. Taylor, Jr., ed., *The Recruitment of Talent for a Medical
Specialty* (St. Louis: Mosby Co., 1961), p. 130; p. 13; p. 134.

37 Ibid., p. 29; p. 134; p. 35; p. 94; p. 134.

38 Ibid., p. 80.

39 Elinor Black, pocket diary, November 13, 1964.

40 Andison, after-dinner speech, November 13, 1964.

41 Letter from Lillias Cringan-MacIntyre to Elinor Black, December 18,
n.d.

42 Dr. Agnes Bishop was appointed head of the Department of Paediatrics
at the University of Manitoba in 1985.

43 Letter from W.J. Condo to Elinor Black, August 27, 1964.

44 Elinor Black, pocket diary, September 1, 1964.

45 Letter from Elinor Black to W.J. Condo, September 10, 1964.

46 Letter from Eva Macfarlane to Elinor Black, Sunday. (Elinor later added "Sept/64.")

47 Elinor Black, pocket diary, September 6, 1964.

48 Ibid., August 7-26, 1962.

49 Letter from Elinor Black to Jack Pickersgill, August 18, 1965.

50 Letter from Paul Martin to Jules Leger, October 1, 1965.

51 Letters from Elinor Black to Charlotte Black and Marjorie Black, Sydney, March 19, 1966; Florence, June 11, 1966.

52 Ibid., Nagaya, April 3, 1966; Sydney, March 19, 1966.

53 Ibid., March 19, 1966.

54 Ibid., Rome, June 8, 1966.

55 Elinor Black, "The Mouse," story/memoir, unpublished, undated, p. 2.

56 Letter from Elinor Black to Charlotte Black and Marjorie Black, New Zealand, February 9, 1966.

57 Elinor Black, "Mouse," p. 4.

58 Elinor Black, pocket diary, May 31, 1967.

59 *Globe and Mail* (July 1, 1967):A10.

60 Letter from Elinor Black to Ethel, April 10, 1967.

61 R.L. Perkin, M.D., "Medical Manpower in General Practice," *CMAJ*, vol. 97 (December 23, 1967):1,572.

62 I.W. Bean, M.D., "Future Manpower Needs in General Practice," *CMAJ*, vol. 97 (December 23, 1967):1,574-1,577.

63 Elinor Black, *CMAJ*, vol. 98 (March 16, 1968):560.

64 Letters from Elinor Black to V.A. Lindabury, editor, *The Canadian Nurse* (October 19, 1968); (December 13, 1968).

65 Letter from Elinor Black to Helen K. Mussallem, October 19, 1968; letter from Helen K. Mussallem to Elinor Black, October 24, 1968.

66 Letter from Elinor Black to Mervyn Roulston, M.D., Winnipeg, May 25, 1968; letter from Mervyn Roulston, M.D., to Elinor Black, October 23, 1967.

67 Letter from Arthur F.W. Peart, M.D., to Elinor Black, Toronto, July 11, 1967.

68 Elinor Black, pocket diary, April 25, 1968; November 12, 1968.

69 Ibid., throughout 1968.

70 *CMAJ*, vol. 98 (March 16, 1968):560.

71 Letter from Charlotte Black to Elinor Black, October 1, 1968.

72 Letter from A.D. Kelly, M.D., to Elinor Black, Toronto, October 23, 1968.

73 Letter from David B. Stewart, M.D., to Elinor Black, Kingston, November 27, 1968.

74 Ibid., December 22, 1968.

75 Dr. U.N. Pathak, interviewed by author, October 4, 1988.

76 Letter from Elinor Black to A.D. Kelly, M.D., Kingston, March 30, 1969.

77 Elinor Black, pocket diary, January 14, 1969.

78 Pathak interview.

Chapter Twelve: Damn *the Passing Years*

Letter from Elinor Black to Alex Andison, M.D., February 10, 1976.

1 Elinor Black, pocket diary, May 28, 1969; July 1, 1969; May 28, 1969; May 31, 1969.

2 Letter from Elinor Black to Jim Garner, August 31, 1976.

3 Elinor Black, pocket diary, February 21, 1970.

4 Letter from Elinor Black to A.D. Kelly, M.D., February 2, 1967.

5 Ibid.

6 Elinor Black, pocket diary, October 30, 1969; October 8, 1969.

7 Letter from Elinor Black to Jim Garner, August 31, 1976.

8 Elinor Black, pocket diary, March 17, 1970; March 18, 1970; May 5, 1970.

9 Letter from Charlotte Black to Elinor Black, March 18, 1970.

10 Elinor Black, pocket diary, August 2, 1971; August 28, 1971.

11 Letter from Elinor Black to Alex Andison, M.D., dated only 1976.

12 Ibid., April 29, 1975.

13 Ibid., November 5, 1977.

14 Ibid., September 16, 1979.

15 Ibid., undated, 1979; July 3, 1977; September 16, 1979.

16 Letter from Alex Andison to Elinor Black, February 5, 1974.

17 Letter from Elinor Black to Gertrude Rutherford, May 16, 1950.

18 Letter from Elinor Black to Alex Andison, M.D., February 10, 1976.

19 Ibid., April 29, 1975.

20 Ibid., April 17, 1976.

21 Letter from Elinor Black to Loeta Black, August 3, 1975.

22 Letter from Reverend Harold Black to author, December 9, 1988.

23 Ibid.

24 Letter from Elinor Black to Loeta Black, February 5, 1978.

25 Letter from Elinor Black to Alex Andison, M.D., July 3, 1977.

26 Ibid., August 5, 1978.

27 Elinor Black, pocket diary, August 12-13, 1977; January 20, 1978; August 19, 1978.

28 Letter from Elinor Black to Alex Andison, M.D., April 27, 1979; July 29, 1979.

29 Elinor Black, pocket diary, April 22, 1978. Dr. John Tyson was head of obstetrics and gynaecology at the University of Manitoba from 1978 to 1983.

30 Letter from Elinor Black to Alex Andison, M.D., August 7, 1980.

31 Ibid., June 5, 1981. For a current exploration of some of the questions surrounding neonatal technology, see Kerry Banks, "Born Too Soon," *Equinox*, no. 45 (May/June 1989):83-100.

32 Letter from Elinor Black to Alex Andison, M.D., November 27, 1977.

33 Ibid., August 13, 1981.

34 Ibid., January 3, 1982.

35 Letter from Alex Andison, M.D., Markham, to Elinor Black, January 15, 1982.

36 Letter from Elinor Black to Alex Andison, January 20, 1982.

37 Cosbie, *History*, p. 25.

38 Sir William Fletcher Shaw, "The College: Its Past, Present and Future," *The Journal of Obstetrics and Gynaecology of the British Empire*, no. 4 (August 1954):558.

39 *The Lancet* (April 14, 1979):819.

40 Linda McQuaig, "Doctor's Choice, Mother's Trauma," *Maclean's* (July 28, 1980): 46-47.

41 Andrea Boroff Eagan, "The Estrogen Fix," *Ms.*, April 1989, p. 43.

42 See, McDonnell, Adverse Effects; *D.E.S.: An Uncertain Legacy*; Corea, *The Hidden Malpractice*; Hubbard et al., *Women Look at Biology*; Strother Ratcliff, *Healing Technology*; Lewin and Olesen, *Women, Health and Healing*; and *The New Our Bodies, Ourselves*.

43 Holly Cupert and Dianne Lai, "Long Distance Delivery," *Healthsharing*, vol. 10 (Winter 1988):17. See also Douglas P. Black, M.D., "The Safety of Obstetric Services in Small Communities in Northern Ontario," *CMAJ*, vol. 130 (March 1, 1984):571-576.

44 *The Ottawa Citizen* (June 23, 1988):A23, CP wire service.

Bibliography

Adamson, J.D., M.D. "The Manitoba Medical College, 1883-1958." *The Manitoba Review* 38 (1958).

Allen, Ralph. "You Can't Lick a River That Won't Fight Back." *Maclean's* (July 1, 1950).

Angel, Barbara, and Michael Angel. *Charlotte Whitehead Ross*. Winnipeg: Peguis Publishing Ltd., 1982.

Banks, Kerry. "Born Too Soon." *Equinox* 45 (1989).

Bean, I.W., M.D. "Future Manpower Needs in General Practice." *Canadian Medical Association Journal* 97 (December 23, 1967).

Bellan, Ruben. *Winnipeg First Century: An Economic History*. Winnipeg: Queenston House Publishing Co. Ltd., 1978.

Beynon, Francis Marion. *Aleta Dey*. London: Virago Press, 1988. First published in Great Britain: C.W. Daniel, Ltd., 1919.

Black, Donald M., M.D. "Francis Molison Black 1870-1941" (unpublished), 1966. Provincial Archives of Manitoba.

Black, Douglas P., M.D. "The Safety of Obstetric Services in Small Communities in Northern Ontario. *Canadian Medical Association Journal* 130 (March 1, 1984).

Black, Elinor F., M.D. "A Pi Phi Doctor." *The May Arrow* (May 1936).

_____. "The Use of Testosterone Propionate in Gynaecology." *Canadian Medical Association Journal* (August 1942).

_____. "The Uses and Abuses of Endocrine Therapy." *Manitoba Medical Review* 25 (November 1945).

_____. "Symposium on Caesarian Section." *Manitoba Medical Review* 30 (1950).

_____. "The Treatment of Dysmenorrhoea with Phenylbutazone." *Canadian Medical Association Journal* 79 (November 1, 1958).

_____. "The Obsolescence of Leisure." *Canadian Medical Association Journal* 85 (October 21, 1961).

_____. "Gynaecological Endocrinology." *Manitoba Medical Review* 45 (1965).

_____. "The Professor and His Wife" (unpublished), 1971. Department of Archives and Special Collections, Elizabeth Dafoe Library, University of Manitoba.

_____. "Thinking Back." *Canadian Medical Association Review* 105 (July 1971).

_____. "Not So Long Ago." *University of Manitoba Medical Journal* 45 (1975).

_____. "The Department of Obstetrics and Gynaecology." *University of Manitoba Medical Journal* 51 (1981).

Black, Frank. "Patrick Burns as I Knew Him." *Saturday Night* (March 27, 1937).

Brittain, Vera. *Testament of Friendship.* London: Fontana, 1981.

Callwood, June. "Painless Childbirth — Sometimes." *Maclean's* (July 15, 1950).

Chafe, J.W. *An Apple for the Teacher:* The Winnipeg School Division No. 1, 1967.

Chown, H.B., M.D. "The Story of the Medical College: 'Worship Great Men.'" *University of Manitoba Medical Journal* 5 (1933).

Clarke, Edward H., M.D. *Sex in Education; or, A Fair Chance for the Girls.* Boston: James R. Osgood and Company, 1873. Reprint edition 1972 by Arno Press Inc.

"Close-Up." Canadian Broadcasting Corporation (CBC) Television, November 3, 1957.

Corrigan, C.E., M.D. "Sixty Years of Medicine in Manitoba." *University of Manitoba Medical Journal* 44 (1974).

Cosbie, W.G., M.D. *The History of the Society of Obstetricians and Gynaecologists of Canada*. Published by the Society, 1967.

Cupert, Holly, and Dianne Lai. "Long Distance Delivery." *Healthsharing* 10 (1988).

Dafoe, W.A., M.D. "The Types and Treatment of Abortions." *Canadian Medical Association Journal* (June 1930).

Dick-Read, Grantly, M.D. *Childbirth without Fear: The Original Approach to Natural Childbirth*. Fifth edition. New York: Harper and Row, 1984. The original edition was *Natural Childbirth*, published in 1933 by London, Heinemann.

Dunmire, Jean M. "The Winnipeg Birth Control Society in the 1930s: The Social Reform Lobby for a Healthy Birth Controlled World" (unpublished, 1988). Provincial Archives of Manitoba.

Eagan, Andrea Boroff. "The Estrogen Fix." *Ms.* (April 1989).

"First Fifty Years, 1895-1945: The Training and Work of Women Employed in the Service of the United Church of Canada." Toronto: The United Church of Canada, n.d.

Godfrey, C.M., "Origins of Medical Education of Women in Ontario." *Medical History* 17 (1973).

Goodall, James R., M.D. "Puerperal Infections." *Canadian Medical Association Journal* (May 1930).

Gray, James H. *Red Lights on the Prairies*. Toronto: Macmillan of Canada, 1971.

Hacker, Carlotta. *The Indomitable Lady Doctors*. Toronto: Clarke Irwin, 1974.

Hamilton, Margaret Lillian. *Is Survival a Fact?* London: Psychic Press Ltd., 1969.

Hamilton, T. Glen, M.D. *Intention and Survival*. Toronto: The Macmillan Company of Canada Ltd., 1942.

Holtby, Winifred. *Women and a Changing Civilization*. London: John Lane, The Bodley Head Ltd., 1934.

Hurst, W.D. "The Red River Flood of 1950." Published by the Historical and Scientific Society of Manitoba. Series 3, number 12, 1957.

Klass, Perri, M.D. *A Not Entirely Benign Procedure*. New York: Signet, 1987.

Lawrence Greene, Margaret. *The School of Femininity: A Book for and about Women as They Are Interpreted through Feminine Writers of Yesterday and Today*. Toronto: Musson Book Company, 1972.

MacDonald, Eva Mader, M.D., and Elizabeth M. Webb. "A Survey of Women Physicians in Canada, 1883-1964." *Canadian Medical Association Journal* 94 (1966).

MacMurchy, Helen, M.D. *Sterilization? Birth Control?* Toronto: The Macmillan Company of Canada Ltd., 1934.

Margolese, M. Sidney, M.D. "The Diagnosis and Treatment of the Climacteric." *Manitoba Medical Review* 24 (April 1944).

"Maternal Mortality." *Manitoba Medical Bulletin* 78 (February 1928).

McGeachy, Jessica, M.D. "A Career in Obstetrics and Gynaecology." *Ontario Medical Review* 19 (1952).

McQuaig, Linda. "Doctor's Choice, Mother's Trauma." *Maclean's* (July 28, 1980).

Medovy, Harry, M.D. *A Vision Fulfilled: The Story of the Children's Hospital of Winnipeg, 1909-1973*. Winnipeg: Peguis Publishers Ltd., 1979.

Mitchell, Ross, M.D. *Medicine in Manitoba: The Story of its Beginnings*. Winnipeg: The Manitoba Medical Association, 1955.

_____. "Maternity Hospitals of Greater Winnipeg." *Manitoba Medical Review* 26 (1946).

"News Items." *Manitoba Medical Association Review* (October 1937).

Parsons, Alice Harriet. "Careers or Marriage?" *Canadian Home Journal* (June 1938).

Perkin, R.L., M.D. "Medical Manpower in General Practice." *Canadian Medical Association Journal* 97 (December 23, 1967).

Pickersgill, J.W. *My Years with Louis St. Laurent.* Toronto: University of Toronto Press, 1975.

Rasky, Frank. *Great Canadian Disasters.* Toronto: Longmans Green and Company, 1961.

"Safeguarding Motherhood: The Winnipeg General Hospital Maternity Wards 1888-1950." Winnipeg: The Board of Trustees of the Winnipeg General Hospital, n.d.

Shaw, Sir William Fletcher. "The College: Its Past, Present and Future." *The Journal of Obstetrics and Gynaecology of the British Empire* 4 (August 1954).

"Should Women Earn Pin Money?" *Maclean's* (April 1, 1930).

"The South London Hospital for Women and Children." London: published by the Amenity Fund, March 1966.

Spencer, Steven M. "Do Women Make Good Doctors?" *Saturday Evening Post* (November 13, 1948).

Stassinopoulos, Arianna. *The Gods of Greece.* Toronto: McClelland and Stewart, 1983.

"Survey of Illness amongst Unemployed in the City of Winnipeg." *Manitoba Medical Association Review* (February 1937).

Taylor, Jr., Howard C., ed. *The Recruitment of Talent for a Medical Speciality.* Saint Louis: C.V. Mosby Co., 1961.

Todd, Margaret Georgina. *The life of Sophia Jex-Blake.* London: Macmillan and Company Ltd., 1918.

Willson, Robert J., M.D., and Elsie Reid Carrington, M.D. *Obstetrics and Gynecology*. Seventh edition. St. Louis: The C.V. Mosby Company, 1983.

"Women in Medicine." *The Canadian Doctor* (April 1936).

Index